M000207254

The Microbiome Diet Reset

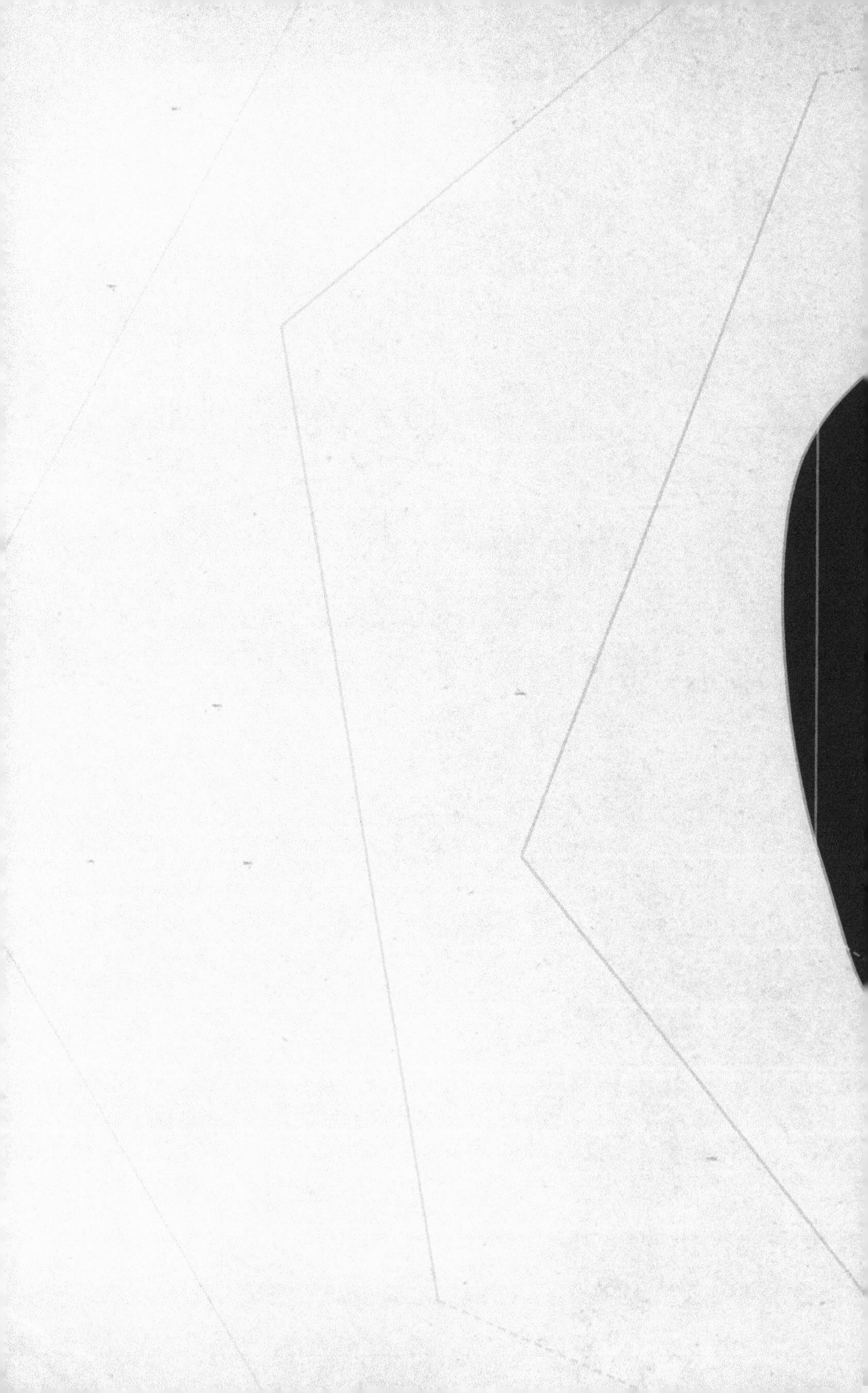

THE Microbiome Diet Reset

A Practical Guide to Restore and Protect a Healthy Microbiome

MARY PURDY, MS, RDN

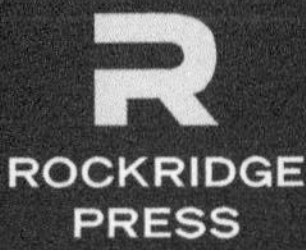

Copyright © 2020 by Rockridge Press, Emeryville, California

No part of this publication may be reproduced, stored in a retrieval system, or transmitted in any form or by any means, electronic, mechanical, photocopying, recording, scanning, or otherwise, except as permitted under Sections 107 or 108 of the 1976 United States Copyright Act, without the prior written permission of the Publisher. Requests to the Publisher for permission should be addressed to the Permissions Department, Rockridge Press, 6005 Shellmound Street, Suite 175, Emeryville, CA 94608.

Limit of Liability/Disclaimer of Warranty: The Publisher and the author make no representations or warranties with respect to the accuracy or completeness of the contents of this work and specifically disclaim all warranties, including without limitation warranties of fitness for a particular purpose. No warranty may be created or extended by sales or promotional materials. The advice and strategies contained herein may not be suitable for every situation. This work is sold with the understanding that the Publisher is not engaged in rendering medical, legal, or other professional advice or services. If professional assistance is required, the services of a competent professional person should be sought. Neither the Publisher nor the author shall be liable for damages arising herefrom. The fact that an individual, organization, or website is referred to in this work as a citation and/or potential source of further information does not mean that the author or the Publisher endorses the information the individual, organization, or website may provide or recommendations they/it may make. Further, readers should be aware that websites listed in this work may have changed or disappeared between when this work was written and when it is read.

For general information on our other products and services or to obtain technical support, please contact our Customer Care Department within the United States at (866) 744-2665, or outside the United States at (510) 253-0500.

Rockridge Press publishes its books in a variety of electronic and print formats. Some content that appears in print may not be available in electronic books, and vice versa.

TRADEMARKS: Rockridge Press and the Rockridge Press logo are trademarks or registered trademarks of Callisto Media Inc. and/or its affiliates, in the United States and other countries, and may not be used without written permission. All other trademarks are the property of their respective owners. Rockridge Press is not associated with any product or vendor mentioned in this book.

Interior and Cover Designer: John Calmeyer
Art Producer: Sue Bischofberger
Editor: Gurvinder Singh Gandu
Production Editor: Rachel Taenzler

Illustration © 2019 Leonardo Gauna

Cover Photography © Alicia Cho, Biz Jones, Emulsion Studio, Marija Vidal, Marcus Spiske/Unsplash, Floortje/iStock, eriksvoboda/iStock, Azure-Dragon/iStock, Igor Sirbu/Shutterstock, sabyna75/Shutterstock, and spline_x/Shutterstock.

Interior Photography © Foxys Forest Manufacture/shutterstock, p. vi; Alessio Bogani/Stocksy, p. 2; Harald Walker/Stocksy, pp. 10-11, 40-41, 61, and 112-113; Ina Peters/Stocksy, p. 16; Elysa Weitala, p. 24; Sara Remington/Stocksy, p. 26; Emulsion Studio, pp. 48 and 104; Shebeko/Shutterstock, p. 62; Dobránska Renáta/Stocksy, p. 90; Darren Muir, p. 92; Rowena Naylor/Stocksy, p. 98; Alexander Grabchilev/Stocksy, p. 106; Sharon McCutcheon/Unsplash, p. 116; Andrew Purcell, p. 128. Author photo courtesy of Autumn Azure.

ISBN: Print 978-1-64152-532-9
eBook 978-1-64152-533-6

R0

For my partner in life, Keith, and for the trillions of microorganisms in my own gut that have kept me healthy and happy over many years. And for the curious and stubborn two-year-old Mary Purdy, who for some unknown reason decided to lick the floor of the airport in Kabul, Afghanistan, which has likely fortified my gut for a lifetime.

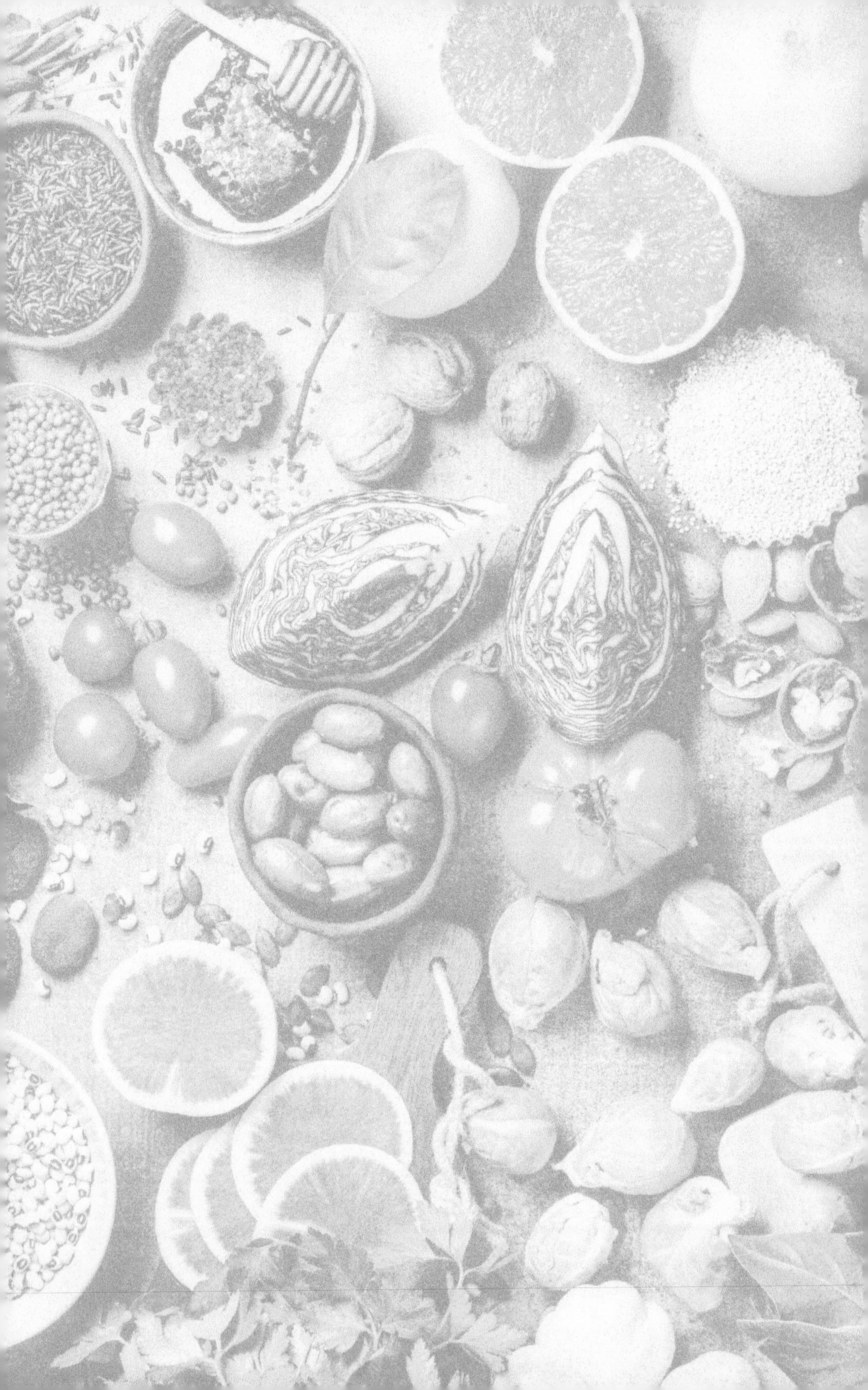

Contents

Introduction

As a dietitian who has been in clinical practice for more than 12 years—one who can genuinely say that she enjoys talking about poop, even at the dinner table—I am thrilled to be providing you with a guide that is easy to navigate, interesting to read, and simple to apply. You may have picked up this book out of sheer curiosity and, if so, welcome! Or maybe you've been struggling with health issues, digestive or otherwise, that just don't seem to resolve, and you're seeking answers—a big hello to you, as well. I hope this book will be helpful, even if it just gives you a better understanding of what may be going on with your digestive function.

I've worked with more than 1,500 patients who have struggled with every health concern you can think of—autoimmune diseases, inflammatory issues, insulin resistance, cardiovascular worries, and obesity, as well as depression, chronic fatigue, fibromyalgia, migraines, and skin problems. While some issues are more serious than others, I've found that most chronic conditions almost always take me back to the body's main hub of wellness: the gut. This is the place, of course, where we digest, absorb, and process our nutrients from the food we eat, but it is also the space where we produce nutrients, communicate with our brain, inform our immune system, detoxify, and eliminate waste.

Time and again, I've found that when I've helped individuals resolve digestive issues or focus on enhancing gut health, many other health problems work themselves out or, at the very least, improve. Currently, many chronic conditions are addressed with medications that suppress symptoms instead of working to get to the root cause of why things got out of balance and stopped functioning properly in the first place. In numerous cases, we can point to dysfunction in the digestive tract as being at least a contributing factor, if not a main culprit, and switching up one's diet and lifestyle can be the key to turning things around. It has been incredibly gratifying to witness people overcome health issues they thought were "just the way things were." This is why I'm delighted to be offering you this book to help you uncover what might be going on and lead you back to a road to vitality.

I've also spent four years working at a company that collected and tested stool samples in order to determine the level of diversity of organisms in the microbiomes of our clients. While working with this organization, I was able to help a number of clients connect the dots between what was happening in their gut and the symptoms they were experiencing, whether related to gastrointestinal (GI) or immune function. In many cases, when they introduced a greater variety of more nutritious foods rich in fiber, removed some of the food aggravators, and modified non-supportive lifestyle habits, we noted a difference in the makeup of their microbial community. In turn, they noticed a difference in how they felt.

You may have heard the phrase, "The way to a man's heart is through his stomach." Well, I'll put my own twist on that and say, "The way to a person's well-being is through their gut." And this book is a perfect place to start, whether you're looking for a few tweaks or a real overhaul aimed at improving your mental, emotional, and physical well-being.

The chapters ahead will provide you with helpful insights into the role these gut bugs play in our lives. They will also offer simple and realistic ways to effectively modify your community of gut bacteria via diet and lifestyle strategies—and to make sure that it's both easy and pleasurable to do so. In my experience, when people enjoy the changes they make, it's a lot more fun to stick to the plan. That's why I have given you a bevy of mouth-watering and fairly simple recipes that you can start incorporating into your diet immediately.

There are also a couple of options for meal plans to suit your needs. You may be the person who's ready to go all out, do a 180, and maybe even throw a dinner party with your soon-to-be new favorite foods. Or you may be that person with the sensitive system who needs to be mindful of what you eat in order to avoid stomach aches and unpleasant GI symptoms. Either way, this book has you covered.

You have a jolly journey ahead. Not only will you be embarking on a crash course into the microbiome, but you will also be given a step-by-step process on how to make changes that give you the biggest bang for your biome buck. You'll be outfitted with lists of foods to include (and how to include them) and foods to avoid (and why), a comprehensive shopping guide, supplement suggestions, meals plans, time-saving tips, and supportive lifestyle strategies, as well as ideas for natural alternatives to household cleaning products, personal care products, and home remedies for common ailments.

Just think of yourself as the newly elected leader of your microbial nation. Your decisions and actions matter and can help turn your kingdom into a thriving community of bacteria, all working together to ultimately serve you and the entire land that is your body. Even simple dietary changes over the next month can set the course for an improved microbiome and a healthier you. How cool is that? Believe me, it's cool, and not just for a gal who enjoys a poop conversation over her arugula salad.

As you read ahead, you may note that I don't use words like "cure," "solve," or "transform." This reset is not meant to give you false hope that miraculous events will occur once you start eating bean salads and cut back on the donuts. It *is* meant to help inform you, empower you, and guide you (and, dare I say, inspire you?) to make some shifts that can support the health of your microbiome. I will tell you this for sure: No one I have ever known, or worked with, who made beneficial changes to their diet hasn't experienced some kind of benefit to their well-being. When the gut is happy, the human is usually happy.

The recommendations made in this book are specific to the microbiome and overall gut health. They are not meant to be strategies for when there may be unusual circumstances or public health issues or crises. It is always a good idea to follow standard hygiene procedures and public health guidelines when necessary, including washing your hands with soap and water, or using hand sanitizer to avoid passing germs on to others.

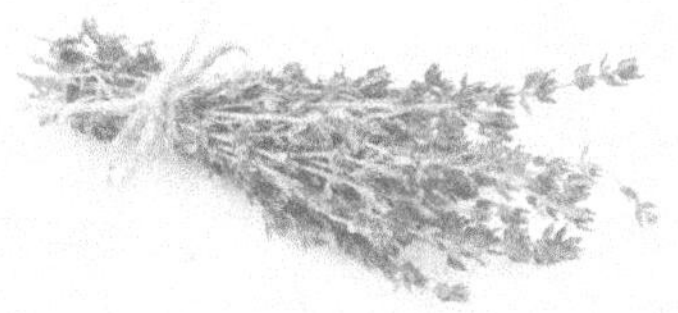

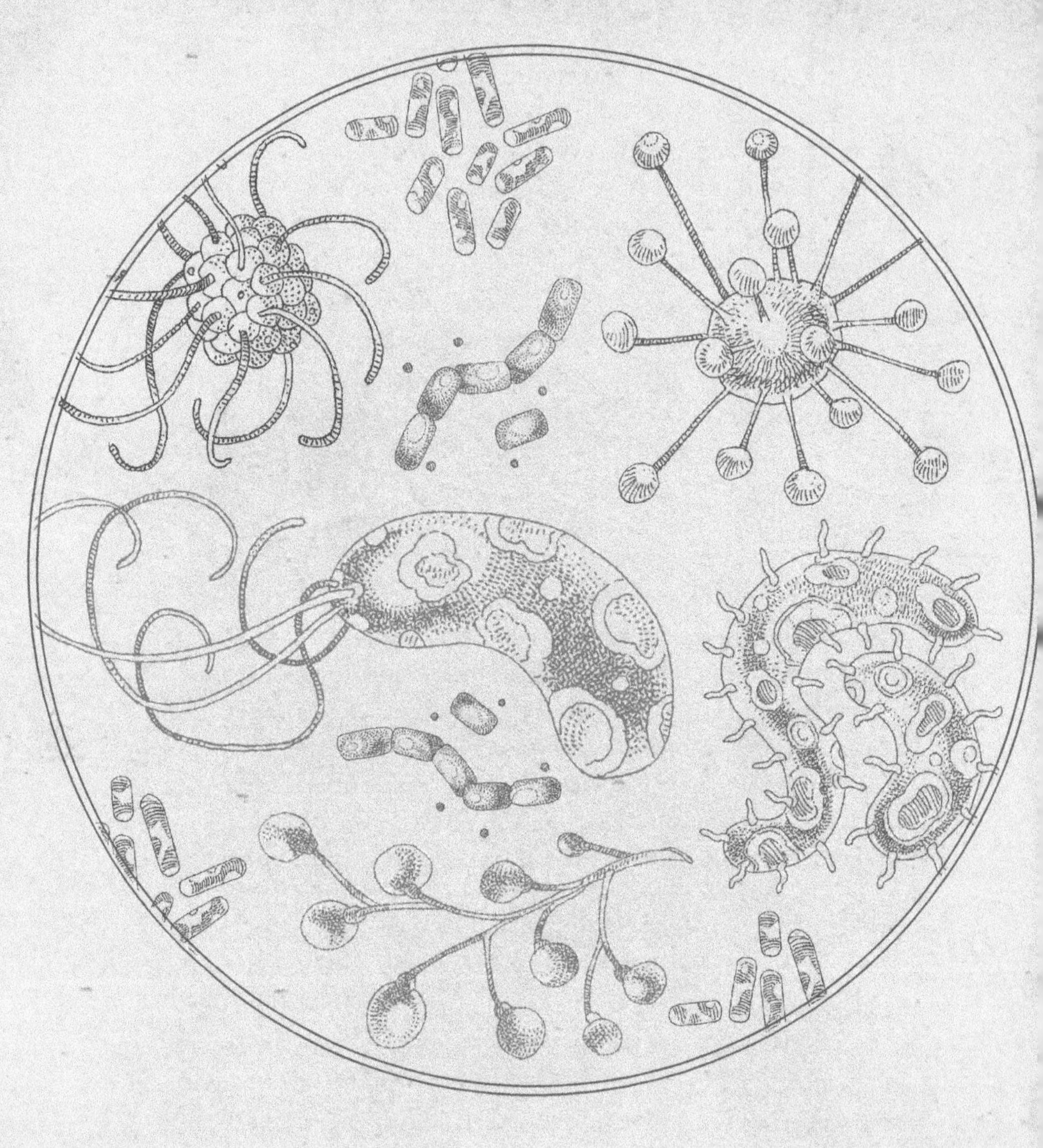

PART ONE

Meet Your Microbiome

ALTHOUGH YOU WERE born with a specific set of microbes in your gut and have been acquiring more along the way throughout your entire life, you may not be very familiar with these residents that you have housed for many years. It's time to finally get to know and begin to better understand their relationship to your health and state of mind. Let the meeting begin!

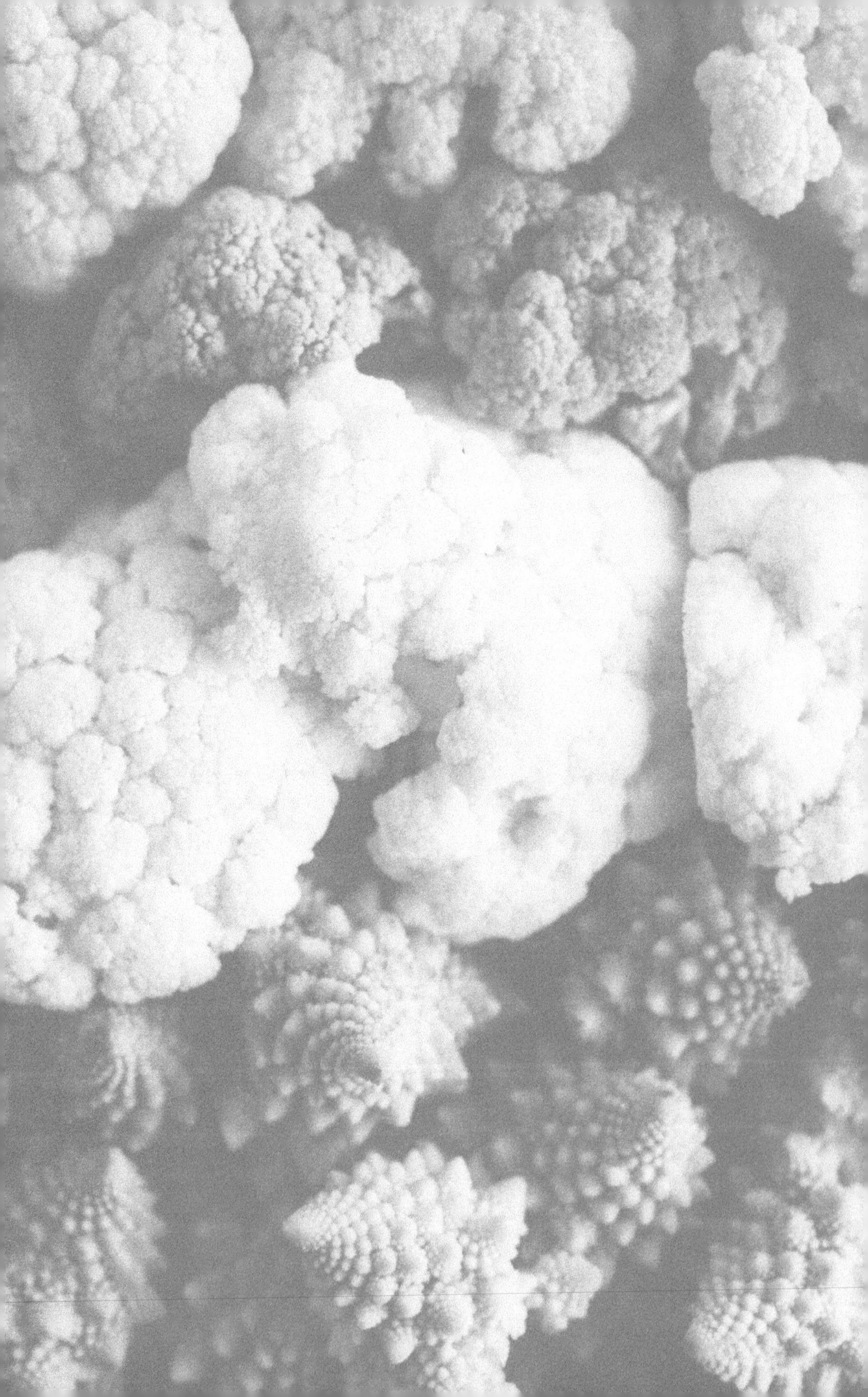

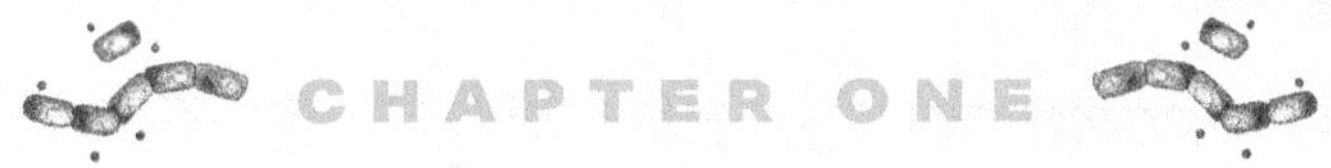

CHAPTER ONE

The Overview

It's hard to read Internet news or peruse the magazine aisles these days without seeing some headline about the microbiome. Research around the microbiome is absolutely exploding. We've known for some time that *how* we digest, absorb, and metabolize our food relies heavily on the status of the bacterial communities within our digestive tract. However, recent scientific developments are proving that the gut has a much greater influence on our overall health than was previously known. The more scientists dive into the topic, the more connections are made between gut health and pretty much every network in the body, including the neurological, cardiovascular, and immune systems. Gut health can even affect our risk of cancer and how well we balance our blood sugar. For many people who have been struggling with confusing health issues, tapping into this wealth of microbiome information has been a place to seek possible answers and find hope.

Your Community of Microbes

"What are microbes?" you may ask. These teeny life-forms—which include bacteria, fungi, and viruses—find homes on or inside our bodies (in the gut, vaginal area, mouth, eyes, and nose, as well as on the skin) and play a significant role in human health. It's easy for bacteria to get a bad reputation (enter the antibacterial cleaning products), but many are quite beneficial and are even necessary for humans to survive and thrive. Collectively, these organisms are called the "microbiota"—formerly called microflora—and when you add their genetic material, it is referred to as the microbiome.

The lower part of the intestinal tract alone is home to between 400 and 500 different species of bacteria, all of which may play a variety of roles in the body, including nutrient digestion, absorption, metabolism, vitamin synthesis, and immune function. These microorganisms also have an impact on how much energy we burn and how much fat we store, playing a vital role in helping us survive. These bacteria tend to reside in the lower bowel area—although some are considered "transient" in that they are just passing through but don't put down any real roots. There tend to be sparse amounts in the stomach and upper intestinal area, although this can shift when an imbalance occurs in the gut.

Then there's our skin, the body's protective barrier, which contains a diverse array of helpful bacteria that provides a first line of defense against harmful bacteria that can cause infection.

Your mouth also has its own little protective ecosystem. Oral bacteria hang out inside our cheeks, on our tongue, and in our gums. While there may be some bad bacteria lurking inside that can cause disease (such as gingivitis), there are also plenty of good microbes acting as guardians of the gums. This is why brushing, flossing, and cutting back on sweets—on which the bad guys thrive—can be helpful for keeping this community balanced. Note that certain mouthwashes that are meant to kill bacteria also rid our mouths of bacteria that we need.

For women, the vaginal area also houses numerous "good" bacteria to keep out the bad ones that can cause yeast infections and urinary tract infections and may lead to an overgrowth called bacterial vaginosis. When babies are born vaginally, they are essentially "colonized" by the bacteria from the vaginal canal. The bacteria set up shop and form the basis for the infant's microbiome, which essentially "educates" the body's immune system to recognize the bacteria as its own. Babies born by C-section—who are more likely to have allergies, asthma, and other health issues—tend to be colonized by the bacteria on the mom's skin instead of that of the birth canal. A new practice called vaginal seeding is occurring more often, whereby the doctor swabs the baby with bacteria from the vaginal area in order to help with optimal colonization of appropriate microbes.

A central point of this book is the concept of bio-individuality, meaning that each of us is unique because of the variety of different factors that have occurred throughout our lives, including the very beginning. It's about much more than just the genes we got from our parents. The distinctive makeup of our personal microbial community can be affected by everything from how we were born (vaginally or by caesarian) and if we were breastfed to where we lived, whether we had pets, whether we took antibiotics frequently, whether we spent time barefoot outdoors, what we ate, what we currently eat, and much more!

As a result, the bacteria hanging out in your gut might be quite unlike those spending time in your best friend's gut because of the differences in your backgrounds, lifestyle, genetics, and food consumption. Numerous studies in the past several years have shown that children and adults in developing countries have a very different makeup of organisms in their guts compared to those in more developed countries, likely due to diverging environmental exposures, sanitation measures, and dietary patterns. Vegetarians, for example, tend to have different bacterial profiles compared to omnivores. All this being said, no matter which bacterial species are currently with us, dietary changes can shift that population for better or for worse.

Everything Is Connected

So, what's the big deal here? How can something so tiny in the gut make such a huge difference in the rest of the body? Well, remember that old song lyric, "The hip bone's connected to the thigh bone"? It's kind of the same with the gut, which is connected to the brain, heart, immune system, and more. A vast amount of research has highlighted the microbiome's role in a variety of conditions, including inflammatory bowel diseases, autoimmune disorders, obesity, depression, autism, Alzheimer's disease, cardiovascular issues, and type 2 diabetes. It seems strange to think that something in your gut might affect something all the way in your brain, but it does. The human body is consistently working in concert with itself in the grand orchestra that is "us," and the microbiome is like the conductor working hard to coordinate all the players so that Beethoven's symphony goes down without a hitch—not an easy task.

First off, the beneficial bacteria in our gut play an integral part in how we digest and break down our food to make it usable as fuel for our bodies. When certain bacteria consume the undigestible parts of the food we eat (fiber and starch found in beans, grains, and some vegetables), they produce both lactic acid, which supports digestion, and something called short-chain fatty acids, which are the main sources of energy for the cells lining your colon. If the community of microbes isn't functioning optimally, or the bad fellas are running out the good fellas, this is going to have an impact on our digestive system. Sometimes, the outcome may just be gas, loose stools, or episodes of constipation. However, when the microbial habitat is disrupted over an extended period of time, individuals can develop "dysbiosis," a severe imbalance and alteration of the organisms in the gut. This can mean less production of short-chain fatty acids and lactic acid, as well as an increase of the bacteria that produce methane and hydrogen associated with several gastrointestinal disorders. In some cases, more serious issues can develop, including irritable bowel syndrome and inflammatory bowel diseases such as Crohn's disease and ulcerative colitis.

But it isn't only about digestive issues. There can be larger implications for the rest of the body. Dysbiosis may also mean less effective or inaccurate signaling to our immune system. Around 60 to 70 percent of our immune system, which protects us from disease, is found in the gut, so the health of our intestines is strongly connected to the overall health of our body. In fact, there is a constant dialogue between our gut microbes and the immune system, which keep each other in check. Part of our immune system works by identifying what is foreign and what is familiar in order to protect us.

One of the ways the gut plays a role here is via a strong and resilient "intestinal barrier," or "gut wall," which keeps microbes and other large molecules from escaping the digestive tract and making their way into the bloodstream. The integrity of this wall relies on the ability of a healthy microbial community nourished by us to create those short-chain fatty acids that nourish the cells of the intestine and strengthen the gut barrier. When the good bacteria go hungry due to lack of sufficient fiber in the diet, they may actually start feeding on the mucosal lining of the intestine as a way to sustain themselves. This, in turn, could compromise the integrity of the gut wall.

Most Americans are significantly lacking fiber in their diets. If that intestinal barrier breaks down as a result of bacterial starvation, imbalances, or ongoing exposure to toxic compounds, foreign bodies are more able to cross from the inside of the intestines to the bloodstream and cause an overactive immune response. There is a strong correlation between this "intestinal permeability" (also known in some circles as "leaky gut") and autoimmune diseases. If you weren't already impressed, these short-chain fatty acids have significant effects on other bodily processes, including supporting healthy cholesterol levels, helping us feel full, potentially increasing calorie burning, and promoting microbial diversity, which keeps the healthy cycle going.

Additionally, there has been a flurry of research regarding what is called "the gut-brain connection." The gastrointestinal tract has often been given the moniker the "second brain" because it is equipped with its own nervous system made up of thousands of neurons. Have you ever had that feeling of butterflies in your stomach? Welcome to your second brain. These gut neurons communicate with those in your brain, and vice versa, via a rather important pathway driven by something called the vagus nerve. Because this "bidirectional" communication affects both emotional and cognitive function, some research suggests that digestive dysfunction is often accompanied by problems with mood and/or cognitive function, or it can put people at a higher risk for these issues.

There are also clear links evolving between a diverse microbiome and an overall effective metabolism. Reduced diversity is correlated with obesity and increased calorie harvesting. Individuals with a less diverse microbiome also tend to have more systemic inflammation (which can be linked to heart, skin, and joint issues), as well as insulin resistance and high cholesterol.

Finally, the gut microbiome is responsible for the synthesis of small amounts of vitamins including biotin, B_{12}, folic acid, thiamine, and vitamin K, all of which play important roles in things like energy production, nerve function, and bone health. If the body is missing out on these nutrients, the physiological processes that rely on them may be affected, particularly if needs are not being met by a well-rounded diet.

Modern Influences on Microbial Life

In many ways, modern life has made our lives more convenient, speedier, and easier to navigate. We have medicines to combat our many ailments, from simple infections to serious illnesses. We wash our clothes with strong detergents, wipe our counters with "powerful" lemon-scented antibacterial spray, swish with fluorescent blue antiseptic mouthwashes, and often breathe in air deodorizers that give us the illusion of evergreen freshness. But these modern conveniences may be coming at a cost to the life of our microbes. In addition to killing off the unwanted bacteria, those sanitizing chemicals, antibiotics, and antibacterial products can wipe out our friendly organisms. Disturbing that bacterial balance can result in negative health effects.

Processed convenience foods are usually lacking in microbe-supportive fiber and nutrients and can be full of chemicals and additives that may further disrupt microbiota function and overall gut health. We frequently eat on the go in a rushed, mindless manner, which can put strain on digestive function. We are also often munching on the same nosh over and over—this lack of diet diversity can translate to a lack of microbial diversity and lowered resilience of our gut bacteria. Much of our soil is depleted of nutrients because of modern agricultural practices, which overuse the land and disrupt the beneficial microorganisms in the ground. According to the Rodale Institute, pesticide residue on produce may be adversely affecting our internal critters, as well. On top of that, we live in more sterilized environments that reduce our exposure to natural dirt and harmless bacteria, and we are quick to wash ourselves clean of bacteria that may actually be serving and protecting us. (Did you know that kids who grow up on farms and with animals are less likely to develop asthma?)

Ironically, with many of these modern developments, we can sometimes find ourselves more stressed, anxious, and less active. All of that can have an impact on the health of our bacteria and can lead to less healthy food and lifestyle choices. This is not to put any blame on you or to bash the many modern comforts we are privileged to have access to. This is more about creating awareness around the potential effects of these conveniences and highlighting the ways a reset can help you get back to simpler diet and lifestyle habits that may be beneficial. There are many natural and healthier alternatives to the potentially harmful commercial products that are out there (see chapter 9). Hundreds of organizations and farmers are currently working on more sustainable farming practices. There are all sorts of whole foods just waiting to be discovered and consumed by you. That's why you picked up this book, right?

Why We Need Healthy Gut Bacteria

By now, you're beginning to recognize how important it is that your community of microbes is happy and healthy in order to keep *you* happy and healthy. If you're still scratching your head about it all, I invite you into my private practice from a few years back for a little story.

SEPARATING HYPE FROM REALITY

Before you start building an altar to a certain probiotic species you've heard about, I want to give you a reality check. It's easy to get pumped about the latest research regarding the microbiome, especially as headlines blast us with the latest hype about how fixing your microbiome will suddenly turn you into "Happy-Pants Peter" or "Skinny-Jeans Jenny." There is a notion that if we "fix the gut," we solve all of our problems and health issues and prevent any potential diseases. As mentioned throughout this book, there is no doubt that better digestion via improving microbiome status has an overall positive effect on our well-being, but how we each get there isn't yet clear.

The emerging science around the microbiome is still being interpreted and understood. While there have been hundreds of animal studies, there simply haven't been enough human studies to provide definitive claims and recommendations, especially when there are numerous factors to consider for each individual. As a result, a lot of the research suggests that these connections that have been made in animals may exist for humans. However, exactly which diseases, which effects, which probiotic species, how much, and for whom are still very much being explored. In most cases, at least currently, we cannot extrapolate that a certain aspect of the gut microbiome has a definite effect on health for all. There are also really no cure-alls or sure things, although advertisers might have you believe otherwise. For instance, the fermented beverage kombucha is regularly touted as being able to transform your gut into a heavenly haven of happy bacteria, bringing you digestive divinity forever. Believe me, I'm a kombucha fan, but one can't rely only on this fizzy beverage to solve all intestinal woes. The same is true for certain probiotic supplements, which, yes, can help digestive function but may offer very little benefit if diet and lifestyle habits aren't also shifting in a more supportive direction.

Additionally, microbiome research is often based on what are called "observational studies," which are essentially observing that certain individuals with specific health issues or medical conditions have more or less of certain types of bacteria in their gut. But it doesn't necessarily prove that more or fewer of those species will definitely mean an improvement or worsening of said health issue in every individual. The bio-individuality of each of us can often make definitive research regarding the microbiome hard to come by because of the many factors that are playing a role. That being said, all research must begin somewhere. Therefore, I will present the best research available and make recommendations in accordance with years of personal clinical experience. I'll also provide you with ideas about how to make smart and scientifically supported decisions about the various ways to potentially help your gut. No doubt, the evidence will continue to grow over the coming decade—I assure you that I'll be on the edge of my seat.

My patient Stella came to me seeking a remedy for all the gas, bloating, and constipation she was experiencing. Her digestion had "been off" for years, she said, and she thought maybe she had food allergies. After some more in-depth discussions, it turned out she was also struggling with depression, unexplained weight gain, and skin issues—namely acne and eczema—that just didn't seem to resolve. Her diet was fairly low in fiber, fruits, and vegetables and high in processed meats and convenience foods, including diet soda. She had also taken numerous courses of antibiotics for chronic sinus infections. Additionally, she was frequently sick in the winter months. However, she never dreamed there was any kind of connection between her skin issues and her constipation, or that her poor gut function may have had something to do with her stubborn weight, especially when she didn't actually feel like she was overeating.

We began by slowly adding more vegetables, fermented foods, beans, and whole grains to her diet. (She actually agreed to a hearty lentil vegetable soup for breakfast.) Stella went on to replace her sweets with cinnamon-sprinkled baked apples and pears and eventually added more foods with anti-inflammatory properties, such as fatty fish, nuts, and seeds, to her diet. Little by little and over the course of six to eight months, her digestion improved, her cravings went down, her skin settled, her weight decreased, and her mood seemed to lift. She even had a flu-free winter. It sounds like a miracle cure, doesn't it? Not really! It's just some help from our happy gut bacteria that enjoy a little extra attention.

When we have healthy gut bacteria, we are that much closer to achieving optimal health. Inflammation can be quelled, immune function can be more balanced, and feel-good chemicals are more likely to be properly produced and communicated to the brain. The stomach feels satisfied, digestion is smoother, and bowel movements get a lot easier.

The Powerful Role of Diet

Good news: Better health may be closer than you think, and it may all begin with your next meal. What we eat nourishes our beneficial gut bugs, so the more that you are able to consume a wide variety of nutrient-dense, fiber-full, and probiotic-rich foods, the better the chance that you'll serve your gut and your gut, in turn, will serve you. It may surprise you that the human gut microbe population is extremely responsive to dietary changes even in as little as 24 hours. This doesn't mean that health issues will resolve in that amount of time, but it's encouraging to know that a steady diet of whole, unprocessed, and supportive foods may set you on a course for wellness. Please note that, because of the individual variation in the acquired and existing makeup of each person's microbiota, there may be different levels of responsiveness to dietary changes. It will very much depend on someone's microbial baseline and other lifestyle and environmental factors that may be having an effect.

One thing that is known for certain is that good bacteria thrive on fiber, which they use to produce those helpful substances like lactic acid and short-chain fatty acids that support our health. So, adding more plant-based foods, including beans, whole grains, nuts, seeds, and brightly colored fruits and vegetables, to your diet is a great way to ensure your bugs are getting what they need to fulfill their functions. Additionally, beneficial plant chemicals called phytochemicals—found in foods like carrots, broccoli, and blueberries—are also friends to our microbiome and can help bugs be more effective in their workplace. When the good guys thrive, it means they not only have the ability to better burn your calories and support your metabolism, but they also have greater power to fight off infection and beat out the bad guys for food.

The world's largest study on human bacteria, the American Gut Project indicated in 2018 that increasing the number of plant foods in the diet (specifically, more than 30 types of plants weekly) increases diversity in the microbial population. This is a good thing since, as mentioned earlier, the more diverse our internal ecosystem is, the more likely we are to be resilient against infection and invaders. Are you a wine lover? A recent human study done in the United Kingdom showed that both regular and occasional red wine consumption was correlated with greater diversity in the microbiome. Do you want to see your microbiome shift? Think of the Mediterranean diet with a fermented flair.

Flipping that coin for a moment, what you *don't* eat is equally as important as what you *do* eat. A diet high in chemicalized and animal foods, processed fats, and refined carbohydrates (sugar, floury foods, chips) has been associated with a reduction in beneficial bacteria and can also feed the less favorable bacteria in the gut. Certain bacteria that flourish with a high intake of red meat (pork and beef) have been associated with lower levels of helpful short-chain fatty acids and with high levels of an unhealthy compound called trimethylamine N-oxide (or the more palatable "TMAO") found in the bloodstream that can increase the risk for heart disease. That doesn't mean red meat is completely off the table—just that portions should be small and consumption less frequent, especially if heart disease runs in your family or you have other risk factors like unhealthy cholesterol levels.

So, it's not just about bringing the supportive sustenance in; it's about minimizing the foods that offer little benefit and, in some cases, may make things worse. It can be hard to completely eliminate certain food groups, especially at first if they are a big part of your habitual patterns, culture, and identity. But as long as you are incorporating more of the aforementioned beneficial foods, you are likely to have a better balance of the helpful bacteria in your gut. Let the adventure begin!

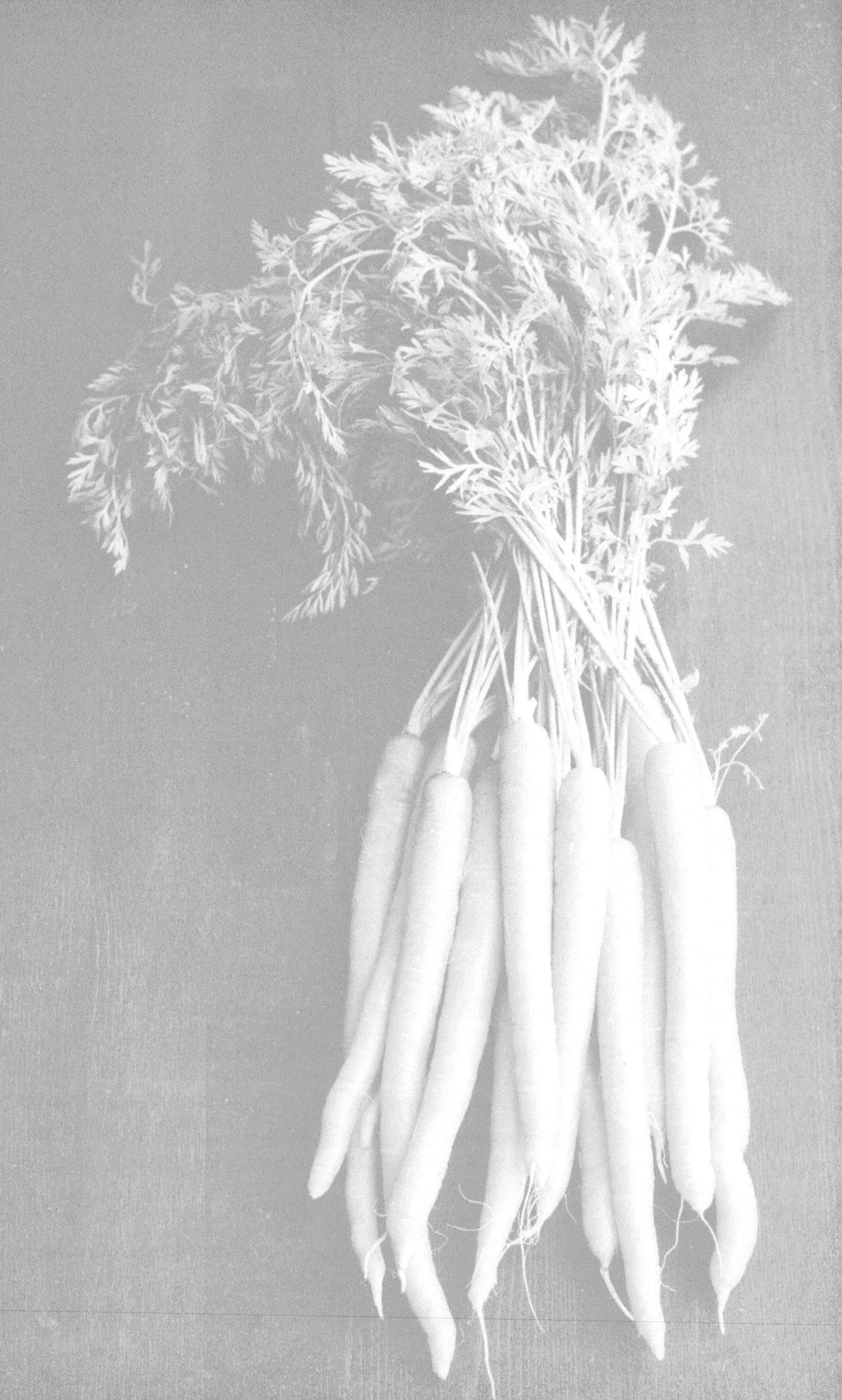

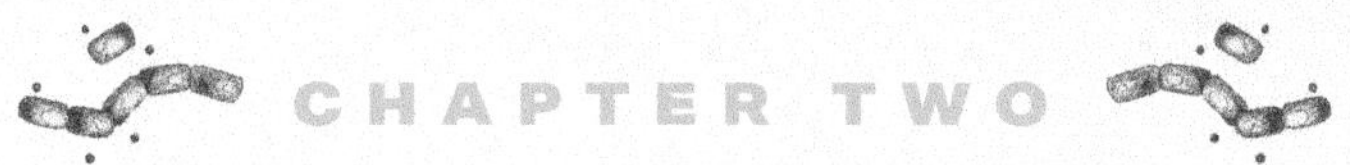

CHAPTER TWO

The Reset

You may be thinking how complicated this all sounds and whether or not you can really do it. Well, here's more good news: This reset is meant for you. While it's not as easy as pressing a button, this guide is meant to take any difficult guesswork and hair pulling out of the process.

The *why* may be clearer at this point, but it's the *how* that you may need to come to terms with—and I promise, it's easier than you think. There's no need to rush into it, pull a 180, and expect yourself to be someone you aren't. Change can take time, so you're welcome to spend a while in prep and contemplation mode and make gradual and realistic shifts. The goal of this reset is to help you keep it simple by giving you easy-to-follow steps that aim to provide your microbiome with the verve it needs to give you the vigor and vitality you seek.

Microbial Resilience

All right. Motivated? Check. Gung ho? Check. And then . . . you enter your kitchen. "Uh oh," you mumble to yourself, eyeing the Cheetos on the counter. "Am I going to just undo all the work of resetting my intestinal ecosystem with a few bites of this alluring cheesy snack?" Not to worry. One bag of chips, a pint of beer, or a slice of birthday cake periodically are not going to unravel the efforts that you make on this reset. Luckily, the microbiome responds well to supportive dietary changes, sometimes quite quickly, as I mentioned earlier. As long as your eating habits are fairly consistent in maintaining the recommendations and guidelines that are laid out here for you, your body should be fairly resilient to less supportive habits every once in a while. While this isn't an invitation to stock up on Pirate's Booty or indulge at every birthday party, it is a reminder that the big picture is what matters. If you're minimizing refined, processed fats and sugars and are regularly consuming fiber, a variety of vegetables, and probiotic-rich food sources, your microbes will continue to thrive and serve you well in the digestive department, as well as work to enhance your immune system, brain, and overall health.

This may take time at first. It's contingent upon where you are with your current dietary patterns and habits. It's also about what you are used to; what you are willing to take on, add, and remove; and in what time frame. Finally, it depends on the current status of the particular bacterial bunch in your gut and whether you have been struggling with digestive distress and other health issues for a long time.

For some, a turnaround in gut microbes may take just a few months. For others, who may have dysbiosis (that imbalance of good and bad microbes) or more significant digestive dysfunction, it can be a longer process. This is especially true if there is an abundance of the bad offenders, and a great deal of damage has been done as a result of less optimal dietary and lifestyle habits. This kind of overhaul may take up to a year for certain people, particularly if stress is high (yes, stress affects our gut bugs, too!) and dietary changes are less consistent.

But this reset is here to help you improve your health and stay resilient. Certain foods not only provide us with good bacteria (probiotics), but they also feed these beneficial bacteria with fiber-rich fuel to run on (called prebiotics).

There may also be a bit of extra gut repair and healing work that needs to be done for those who have a high level of intestinal inflammation. This could require supportive supplementation, such as with high-dose probiotics, digestive enzymes, zinc, and glutamine, which can provide the body with therapeutic compounds that nourish and soothe the intestinal environment and restore intestinal barrier function and strength. (For more on this, see the supplemental section on page 42.)

Fortunately, while the changes in diet and lifestyle can seem like a lot of hard work, the benefits that you may feel as a result can motivate you to keep going. When you feel better, you usually want to continue the healthier habits that got you there. Your body is excellent at giving you feedback, so it is necessary to tune in. You might even find that the bag of Cheetos winking at you from your pantry isn't quite as irresistible as you thought.

You may also need to just stick with it. One step forward and two steps back is often the process of change—just keep ensuring that you're taking that one step forward.

The Two-Step Reset

Flashy headlines and ever-conflicting information about the microbiome and surefire ways to achieve an ideal microbial habitat can be overwhelming, but it doesn't have to be overly complicated. In the end there are only two things you really need to do to help your microbiome thrive. Here's a simple mantra that you can follow in the coming weeks, months, and years: "I will feed my beneficial bacteria and protect and preserve my microbial diversity." Feed, protect and preserve. It's kind of like being on the microbiome task force.

STEP 1
FEED BENEFICIAL BACTERIA

The main goal is to tip the balance in favor of the good bacteria. What does it mean to feed those beneficial bugs? Well, they love fiber and resistant starches, so ensuring that you are taking in fiber daily is going to be key. This is not about downing your grandma's Metamucil and calling it a day—foods in their most whole form are the most nutritious sources. With every bite of fiber-rich vegetables, fruits, nuts, legumes, and fermented foods, we make our bacterial army of soldiers stronger, helping them lord over the bad bacteria.

As noted earlier, most Americans tend to get insufficient amounts of fiber, so knowing your fiber sources is critical. (If you see something in your meal that could potentially get stuck in your teeth, that's a good start.) Here are some good sources of fiber:

- ½ cup beans = 7 grams of fiber
- ½ medium avocado = 7 grams of fiber
- 1 cup whole grains = 4 grams of fiber

Combine those in one dish and you're close to 20 grams of fiber—and we haven't even invited any other vegetables to the party. I smell a hearty grain bowl coming on.

Some emerging research has also found that sugars in mushrooms and grains (like oats or barley) called beta-glucans have both immune-building and prebiotic properties that protect the gut lining and enhance the growth of some of our bacterial buddies. It's pretty easy to enjoy a bowl of oatmeal or toss some fabulous fungi in your salad periodically. As an added benefit, consumption of beta-glucans has also been linked to lower cholesterol levels.

Finally, the inclusion of micronutrients called polyphenols, which are protective plant compounds/phytochemicals, has been shown to inhibit the growth of pathogenic bacteria, stimulate beneficial bacteria, and reduce inflammation in the gut. Plants naturally contain these compounds—often denoted by their vibrant color, which is a way to fend off invaders and predators—and we get the benefits when we eat them. Think of the verdant green in a spinach leaf, the ruby red in a tomato, and the purple hue of a blackberry. Whenever you can, make that plate as polychromatic as possible!

STEP 2

PROTECT AND PRESERVE MICROBIAL DIVERSITY

A high-fiber diet helps nourish our bugs, but it also ensures microbial diversity. The prebiotics found in the foods listed in step 1 (see page 19) are a great way to bring a variety of gut bugs to your colonic jamboree.

Variety in your diet is also imperative. It is, in fact, the spice of life for your bacteria! So, don't get too stuck on only one type of vegetable, one kind of nut, or one class of grains. Try some fennel. Have a hazelnut. Branch out to buckwheat. Diversity of diet equals diversity of microbiome, which equals a happier, healthier you. Shoot for an array of color and texture and a mixture of foods each day that provide both fiber and a plethora of polyphenols, and your bugs will likely sing.

This process is also about doing what you can to avoid unintentionally killing off the good guys. Aside from starving them of nourishment, your exposure to a variety of potentially harmful agents may put them at risk of an early demise. Some of the obvious ones include antibiotics, which are often overused and are quick to knock out our good microbes as they knock out our bad ones. Fortifying your immune system naturally with sufficient protein and brightly colored protective plant foods, herbs, and spices may reduce the frequency with which you need such medications. (For more on this, see chapter 7.)

We also aren't the only ones being prescribed antibiotics. Some of the animals whose meats we consume also get a dose, which means we get microdoses that can add up over time. Studies show that livestock raised organically without antibiotics may have a better effect on our microbiome status. Depending on the farmer, this may also mean that we are supporting more humane and environmentally friendly practices. When possible, seek out organic meat and substitute plant-based meals for meat a couple of times per week, or combine them. Chili, anyone?

There are a number of other commonly prescribed or over-the-counter medications that play a role in our microbial health. Acid blockers, like Tagamet and Prilosec—meant to address acid reflux—can reduce our levels of stomach acid, which acts as a natural defender against bacterial infections. Without sufficient amounts of this key substance in our gut, the bad guys are more likely to enter, take over, and starve out the good bugs. Other medications that may get in the way of a healthy gut include laxatives and NSAIDs, as well as prescribed drugs such as antipsychotics and antidepressants. This is not to dissuade you from taking important medication, but more to help you better understand why things may be off in your gut and the impact it may be having on other aspects of your health. (If you struggle with acid reflux, constipation, or inflammatory issues, take a peek at some of our natural-remedy recipes in chapter 9 as potential alternatives.)

According to research done by the National Academies of Sciences, besides being affected by medication, the livelihoods of our good bacteria are also susceptible to environmental chemicals, including the pesticides found in residues on many of the foods we eat and the chlorine found in the water we drink and in which we swim or soak our bodies. In general, if it's meant to kill pests and germs, it's potentially having a deadening effect on our good bacteria as well. Using plain old soap and water and washing for a full 20 seconds can do the job just fine.

Other things you may be inadvertently consuming include heavy metals like lead, arsenic (sometimes found in rice), and mercury (found in large, fatty fish like tuna). Try some of the smaller fish, like sardines and anchovies, which are lower in mercury. They are more versatile than you might think!

One last culprit in altering good bacteria may be the soil in which we grow our food. Healthy soil should be teeming with healthy microorganisms that have a positive impact on the nutrient value of the crop. Historically, most of us interacted with soil as kids and have even knowingly or unknowingly consumed dirt simply because of the residual amounts on unwashed produce. Unfortunately, because of many current agricultural practices—including the use of chemicals, disruptive soil management methods, and a lack of diverse crops being planted—the richness of the soil and its population of microbes has diminished. This can reduce our exposure to beneficial microbes from plants, which may be linked to a reduced biodiversity in our guts.

You may be familiar with the herbicide glyphosate, used to kill bacteria and fungi on plants. Preliminary evidence suggests that it may also be capable of altering the human gut microbiome by reducing some of the beneficial families residing there. Seek out the "organic" label on your next produce purchase at the grocery store, or if you have access to a farmers' market, ask your local farmer about their farming practices. Not everyone can afford to be certified organic, but they may use regenerative agricultural processes that are gentler on the land. Also, be on the lookout for an urban garden in your community, or forage in a nearby park if you have one. Perhaps a neighbor might be willing to part with an overharvest of plums, or it could be time to start your own garden—even if it's on your kitchen windowsill.

What to Expect from the Reset

If you are in excellent health and have a reasonably varied, colorful, and fiber-rich diet, it's possible that you may not notice a huge shift in how you feel on a day-to-day basis during this reset. Initially, there might be a bit more flatulence (that's the bugs digesting your food!) or perhaps smoother or more frequent (but not excessive) bowel movements. However, over the long term, what you may notice is an improvement in your overall immunity, energy, and mood. That said, it may be hard to determine whether these results are from an improvement in your microbiome or simply a result of consuming more nutrient-dense foods. Plus, if you don't have a markedly difficult baseline to begin with, you may not notice as drastic an improvement as someone who is struggling daily with discomfort, depression, or debilitating symptoms from a more significant health condition.

In order to cover our bases, I've laid out a couple of plans on the reset so that you can choose which one might suit your individual needs best. These plans are meant to help you envision what following this reset might be like for you, although you're welcome to "make them your own" as you see fit, whether it's mixing and matching some of the meals or coming up with a similar version. Creativity is welcome.

Do you have a sensitive system? There's a plan especially for you with food options that won't aggravate your stomach.

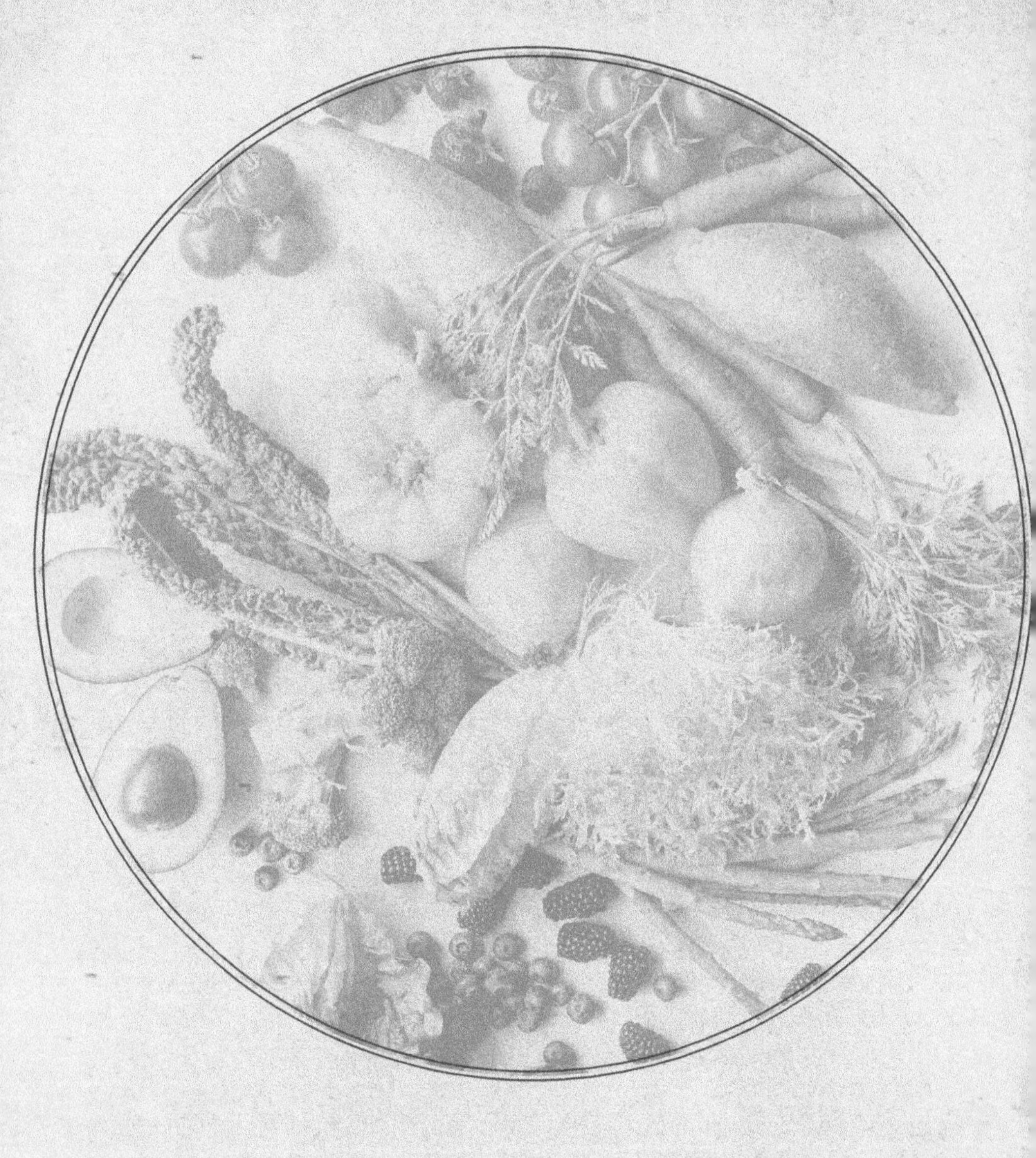

PART TWO

Feed Your Microbiome

OKAY—IF YOU'VE MADE it this far, my guess is you are ready for the plunge. Get out your favorite fork, knife, spoon, bowl, and plate because you're about to embark on a romp through some new gastronomic territory. This is the part you've been waiting for, where I give you ideas about how to eat your way to health, what to avoid, and where to be mindful. You might want to grab a pen as well if you are a note taker, list maker, or word circler. Are you ready to be a super host? Here we go!

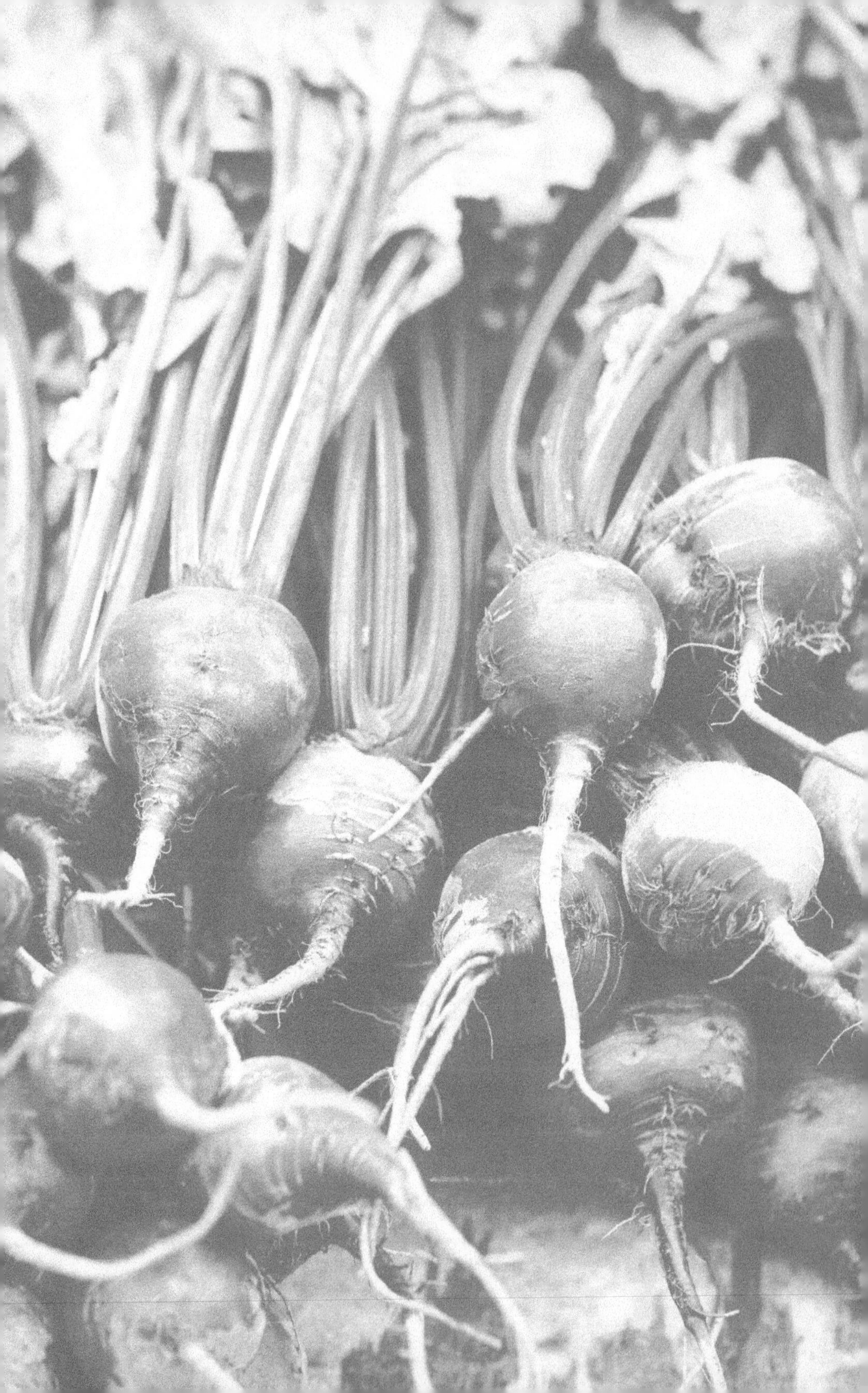

CHAPTER THREE

Guidelines for the Microbiome Diet

Before you hop online to buy the latest and greatest probiotic or other gut health supplement from someone with glowing skin, a flat stomach, and a beaming smile that shouts, "I'm in a fantastic mood!" know that a lot of what you need might be hanging out just a few feet away from you in the refrigerator, pantry, or a hopefully somewhat familiar aisle at your local grocery store or farmers' market. If you subscribe to a "food as medicine" philosophy, like I do, you may believe that removing and replenishing food items is the quintessential first step and perhaps the only step necessary to begin the remodel in your intestinal housing unit. You may prefer to reset your biome without ever opening a bottle besides, say, a bottle of cabernet, kombucha, or beet kvass.

Eat Your Prebiotics

First off, let's talk prebiotics. "Don't you mean *probiotics*, like the stuff in yogurt?" I hear you say. To reiterate, prebiotics are compounds that provide sustenance to the probiotics or good bacteria that we either ingest or already have living in our gut that also need to eat to survive the battle zone in our stomachs. Prebiotics help stimulate growth and diversity of our microbes. Feeding these hungry and beneficial microbes a vast array of fiber bits helps us feel satisfied for longer periods of time and can result in fewer cravings. More important, this is the key to ensuring that all the duties of these good bacteria are carried out, from digestion and metabolism to creating those feel-good chemicals and anti-inflammatory compounds. So, as the prefix "pre" suggests, *before* probiotics can perform their tasks, they need to be properly nourished. (And no, the results after feeding them, such as gas, are not called postbiotics.)

Prebiotics are found in numerous fiber-rich plant foods such as fruits, vegetables, beans, whole grains, nuts, and seeds, and need to be consumed daily. There are foods that contain the specific prebiotic inulin, a soluble fiber found in sprouted wheat, asparagus, garlic, and jicama (and sold as a supplement) that has been shown to nurture the good bacteria. The same goes for another prebiotic found in bananas, leeks, barley, and wheat called fructo-oligosaccharides. That's a mouthful, eh? Also known as "FOS," these prebiotic gems protect against unhealthy bacteria, including those that cause food poisoning.

Foods high in inulin and FOS may actually aggravate the GI symptoms in those with IBS, small intestinal bacterial overgrowth (SIBO), or other digestive issues, so be mindful of how much of these foods you are getting and keep track of symptoms. High intake of such foods is discouraged for those following a low-FODMAP diet (see page 34) or the Sensitive System Meal Plan (see page 55).

Upping these food items alone could have a dramatic impact on the wellness profile of your bacteria. According to the National Academy of Medicine, only about 5 percent of the population is getting the recommended daily amount of fiber, which is 25 grams per day for women and 38 grams per day for men, although numerous schools of thought, including my own, believe this amount may be less than optimal for maximum health benefits for some individuals. The average intake of dietary fiber in the United States is 17 grams per day, which means most Americans are getting half, at best, of what is required for their bacterial population to be nourished properly.

Again, this is not about blame, but rather about how our food system has drastically shifted into the creation of fiber-less convenience foods that can be chewed and swallowed while you're waiting at a red light. A typical bacon, egg, and cheese breakfast sandwich will give you a whopping 1 gram of fiber. That's not a lot, and you only have two more meals and maybe a snack to meet your needs. Be careful about increasing your fiber too rapidly, though, as it can cause a bit of gas due to the stimulation of your bacteria celebrating their expanded food sources. An increase in fiber should also be accompanied by plenty of fluids, otherwise you risk a slowdown in the poop department, which is not super enjoyable.

Starve Less Helpful Bacteria and Other Organisms

It wouldn't be a good story if there weren't a few villains—though, what may be considered villains in one person's body may be bystanders in another. These pathogenic bacteria are, well, let's just say a lot less helpful in that they can cause infection, grow quickly, and compete for food, thus depriving the good bacteria of nourishment. Note that lactic acid has antimicrobial properties that help drive out the bad bacteria, so that's another reason to keep those lactic-acid-producing tribes well fed.

Unfortunately, due to a lack of fiber and a high amount of processed foods in the diet, as well as exposure to medications, chemicals, and food compounds that deplete our good gut microbes, many human intestinal tracts are overrun by these pathogenic inhabitants. Some names of these food crooks may be familiar, like E. coli or C. diff, or less well-known, like Ruminococcaceae. When there is less food available to fortify the good bugs for the bacterial battle, the bad guys inevitably win out in the hunt for fuel. These nefarious creatures tend to thrive on refined carbohydrates like sweetened beverages, confections, and floury goodies (both sweet and savory), so backing off this stuff can be an effective way to starve these bacterial bandits. Research also shows that a diet high in fat tends to be correlated with a higher proportion of the racketeers taking the good stuff from the good guys and using it for their own greedy purposes. High amounts of meat and cheese have also been shown to alter the gut microbiome by helping the bad guys flourish and leading to intestinal inflammation. If you cannot see yourself realistically letting go of meat and cheese completely, see if you can try to at least reduce overall consumption.

One organism that has a voracious appetite for carbs and sugar is not a bacterium but rather a yeast (a type of fungus) called Candida, which, when overgrown, may drive or exacerbate the microbial imbalance in the gut. Healthy bacteria would normally help keep this yeast in check, but if there aren't enough of those in supply, Candida can take charge and cause infections.

So, what's a hungry human to do? Essentially, the goals are to deprive the maleficent microorganisms of the ingredients on which they thrive and to immerse yourself in the world of healthier alternatives so that our helpful residents can use them to your benefit. Love sweet cookies? Try baking with almond flour and using dates for sweetness. Or try replacing the cookies altogether with a handful of some cashews and raisins. Live for chips? Try out some whole-grain crackers instead. Sugar is quite the seducer, but if you eliminate it for a week or two, your taste buds can actually change and things that tasted delicious may start tasting cloyingly sweet. You can also add herbs and spices with natural antibacterial properties—like oregano, rosemary, thyme, cumin, and cinnamon—to your foods, as well as foods like coconut and coconut oil, which have natural antifungal properties. Incorporating these items may help keep the bad guys from winning too easily. Spicy foods can help, too—it's kind of hard to crave sugar when it feels like your tongue is on fire.

Consume Fermented Foods

The long-standing culinary tradition of fermentation originated as a way to preserve food. One of the most common methods of fermentation is to use friendly bacteria to convert sugar into lactic acid, which acts as a preservative. Fermented foods can run the gamut from kimchi to sauerkraut, yogurt, and chutneys. They have been enjoyed in various cultures for centuries and now seem to be having a resurgence as a tangy food with probiotic and health appeal. Having some form of fermented foods daily, if possible, is a definite boon to your body.

Both dairy and non-dairy yogurt that contains probiotics have been shown to reduce the amount of less favorable bacteria in the gut—namely, E. coli and a little fella called Helicobacter pylori (H. pylori), which can be one of the contributors to chronic GI conditions like GERD and even stomach cancer.

When we consume fermented foods, not only are we getting a natural food source of probiotics, but we are also sometimes getting prebiotics in the form of fiber (although this is more the case with fermented vegetables than with yogurt). Additionally, according to a study done in the *International Journal of Food Sciences and Nutrition*, fermentation has been shown to increase the antioxidant activity and availability of the nutrient content of many foods.

That said, not all fermented foods are created equal in terms of their nutritional content. You may be familiar with trusty sauerkraut, which is often an integral part of a hot dog or bratwurst experience. However, many sauerkrauts are pasteurized (heated to high temperatures) in an attempt to improve quality and kill bad bacteria, but this process also kills good bacteria. So, while a pasteurized sauerkraut may be a nice source of fragrant fiber and zingy flavor, it isn't likely to provide the body with much good bacteria.

However, depending on where you live, you may be in luck. All sorts of fermented foods have begun to flood the market. In many places (like the Pacific Northwest, where I live), sauerkraut has taken on a life of its own and comes in a variety of flavors including turmeric, smoky kale, curry, and cumin jalapeño! It's certainly not just your local deli sauerkraut anymore.

If sauerkraut isn't your thing, there are plenty of other options in the fermented vegetable category. One is kimchi, a traditional Korean side dish/condiment of spicy fermented cabbage and other vegetables. If you're unsure exactly how to use it, kimchi can be delicious when mixed with equal parts peanut butter and slathered on whole-grain crackers or as a dip with crudité. Add a little water or coconut milk to the mix and use it as a sauce over rice. If you've ever had a peanut sauce at an Asian restaurant, this will likely taste similar—and all you did was throw two items in your food processor. Other examples include fermented vegetables of all sorts, such as carrots, beets, and cucumbers, although these all need to be raw and unpasteurized.

Contrary to popular belief, if something is pickled, it isn't necessarily fermented—it may just have been made with a ton of salt. There are also fermented condiments, such as salsa and relishes. And if you enjoy slurping your way to gut health in an adventurous manner, I highly recommend beet kvass, a traditional fermented beverage that has a briny zing. It's a bit like sipping the liquid from your sauerkraut jar, which I personally enjoy, but that might not appeal to someone with a sensitive palate or stomach.

But wait, there's more! If fermented vegetables aren't your favorite, you can gain some beneficial bacteria from other fermented food sources, such as the flavorful, curiously popular, and surprisingly expensive fermented drink called kombucha. If you're seeking the 39-cent alternative to the $3.90 bottle of fizz, see my Fauxbucha recipe (see page 103) that uses apple cider vinegar as the fermented base. Miso paste, made from fermented soybeans, is another fabulous option, provided you don't boil it (again, heat kills bacteria). You can mix it with lukewarm water to create a thick paste that can be incorporated into soups after removing them from a strong flame. You can also incorporate it into nut/dried fruit balls for a little salty jazz in a dessert or snack.

Beware of Gut Disruptors

While there are numerous ways that foods can support our gut microbiome, there are also items that we may be consuming that have the potential to disrupt our microbial ecosystem. A higher amount of carbohydrates in general has been associated in some studies with a lower microbial diversity score, although it's important to differentiate between complex carbohydrates, which are higher in fiber, and refined carbohydrates, which are lower. Refined carbs, including high-fructose corn syrup, are among the biggest offenders. This includes not only candy and soda or other sweetened beverages, but also white flour products such as cookies, cakes, crackers, pasta, and scones. That's not to say that you have to totally give up your beloved spaghetti—you might just want to check portions and seek out higher fiber options.

Another potential gut disruptor that may surprise you is artificial sweeteners also known as non-nutritive sweeteners (aka NNS). Although many of these sweeteners are used to reduce calories and help with blood-sugar issues, there are studies showing an association between high consumption of these additives and an increased risk of metabolic syndrome, obesity, and type 2 diabetes.

So what does this have to do with the gut? It turns out that, in certain individuals with diabetes or prediabetes, a reduced ability to properly metabolize sugars (or glucose, the most elemental component of the foods that the body breaks down) can be partially driven by changes in composition and function of the microbiota. Specifically, only saccharin (Sweet'N Low) and sucralose (Splenda) have shown to have this potential effect. Aspartame (Equal) hasn't been shown to have adverse effects on the microbiome, but that doesn't mean it may not come with other potential health risks for some. My advice is to seek out other options for sweetness in your life, including items or activities that aren't food.

Keep an eye out for these ingredients on the nutrition label of the foods and beverages you buy. If you need that added touch of sweetness without the extra calories, you can explore the world of sugar alcohols such as maltitol, lactitol, and xylitol, which may actually help increase some of the good gut bacteria. If it has an "ol" at the end of it, it's an alco-"hol." This means, however, that they are all members of the polyol family, which are on the "avoid list" for anyone working with a low-FODMAP diet. A drop or two of liquid stevia can also be an option periodically, although it is still considered an NNS and its impact on the microbiome is not yet fully understood. A miniscule amount goes a long way.

Finally, emulsifiers—food additives meant to improve the texture and shelf life of certain packaged foods—may also negatively affect the microbiome and increase inflammation, although the research is still emerging and is not conclusive in humans. Examples include carboxymethyl cellulose, polysorbate 80, gum arabic, carrageenan, and arabinogalactan, which you may see in ice creams, salad dressings, alternative milk products, and other commonly consumed items.

I've worked with enough people who find that they don't respond well to these items in their diet, so I think it's worth having a trial separation to see if it benefits your particular issues. Again, it's possible that, for certain individuals, these additives do a whole lot of nothing, but to someone who may be more susceptible, has compromised GI function, and consumes a lot of packaged foods containing these additives, eliminating them may be an excellent idea. One way to avoid these and other additives is to just eat more food in its most natural, unprocessed form—I've got ideas for this, so stay tuned.

Proceed Slowly for Sensitive Systems

Is your brain abuzz with information? Motivation high? Are you about to press hard on the gas pedal? As a special note to my sensitive pals, I'm officially putting up a "proceed slowly" sign right here. Yes, I'm talking to you, person *without* the stomach of steel. If you fall into this category, take a closer look here. People can have sensitive stomachs for a variety of reasons. The one I want to highlight is a lowered ability to digest and break down a family of carbohydrate sugars called FODMAPs. This stands for Fermentable Oligo-, Di-, Monosaccharides And Polyols. This isn't about fermented foods, but rather foods that your bacteria easily ferment.

Certain people will experience symptoms like bloating, gas, diarrhea, and even constipation when these are consumed, especially in large amounts. They can be found in foods like apples, pears, onions, wheat, and dairy and have been shown to cause or worsen symptoms in people with IBS. That doesn't mean you cannot have any of these foods ever. You'll just have to be careful about not going above a certain threshold of the amount that you consume. Long-term adherence to this diet could be problematic because many of these foods are fantastic sources of those obliging prebiotics that feed the probiotics, and fewer of them in the diet could result in reduced diversity.

Microbiome Diet Food Lists

Wondering what you can and cannot eat? Take a look at the following lists so that you know what's on the "Yes," "Not So Much," and "Best to Avoid" lists.

Please note that foods with an asterisk (*) next to them are considered to be in the high FODMAP category and should be consumed in minimal amounts if you know you are sensitive to them. All FODMAP-containing foods are not listed here, but there's an app from Monash University out of Australia that's a fantastic resource for helping you stay on track (see the Resources section).

FOODS TO EAT FREELY

The following are all foods you should feel welcome to eat freely (unless, of course, you know they bother your stomach):

Alliums (Onions, Leeks, Garlic, Scallions): This category of foods, in particular, is an excellent source of prebiotics and can be extremely nourishing to our bugs. If you thought certain foods were lacking in flavor, try sautéing what you think of as that "boring" vegetable or tofu with any member of this family and witness the makeover. Good-quality olive oil, sesame oil, or coconut oil can all help with the transformation of taste.

***Beans, Legumes, and Pulses:** This family of foods is one of the easiest ways to get a high amount of fiber in a small amount of food. You know how beans make some folks a little gassy? That's a by- product of our bacterial buddies chowing down on that chili you just consumed for dinner. Don't get stuck in a bean rut. Seek out your bean aisle or peruse the bulk bin at your local grocery store and see if you can try for three different types of beans each week. Great northern, anyone?

Brightly Colored Fruits and Vegetables: Not only do these gems provide fiber, but they are also filled with polyphenols that increase diversity in the gut and offer anti-inflammatory compounds that are essential for disease prevention and healing. Please note that white and brown are colors in this category—hello, cauliflower, daikon radish, and mushrooms! Good fungi are particularly anti-inflammatory, rich in beta-glucans, and a good source of the immune-supportive vitamin D.

Remember that variety is key here. Just because broccoli gets a special place in the world of superfoods doesn't mean that you should eat only broccoli. Branch out: How about trying bok choy, napa cabbage, or an orange pepper? Include a spectrum of color on your plate and make sure that some of these vegetables are periodically eaten raw or lightly steamed, which may have greater benefits to your microbiome.

Herbs and Spices: Not only incredibly rich in those anti-inflammatory polyphenols, this category of foods also has natural digestive-aid properties that can help improve the digestibility of certain foods like beans. They can also stimulate the production of bile, an essential part of our body's mode of breaking down fat. Plus, they add pizzazz to any meal.

Nuts, Seeds, and Their Respective Butters: This family of foods provides fiber, and it is also a good source of healthy and anti-inflammatory fats that help keep the digestive tract balanced and nourished. It's time to step out of that almond rut and seek out new nutty experiences. Walnuts have been shown to confer excellent benefits on the microbiome because of their high omega-3 and polyphenol content. And if you haven't tasted a buttery hemp seed, also rich in omega-3s and fantastic atop oatmeal, here's your opportunity.

Starchy Vegetables: These hearty vegetables are a great source of fiber and beneficial plant chemicals. When slightly cooled, they are also a source of something called resistant starch, which feeds the bacteria and enables them to create those fantabulous short-chain fatty acids. These include foods like potatoes, winter squash, and root vegetables like parsnips, beets, and rutabaga. When was the last time you munched on rutabaga? This might be your chance!

Teas: This can be green, white, or black tea, all of which contain healthy anti-inflammatory compounds that are beneficial for our microbes and overall gut health. It can also be herbal tea, which is an easy way to add overall health-supportive nutrients to our diet without a lot of additional burden on our digestive system.

Unprocessed Whole Grains: These are wonderful complex carbohydrates (meaning fiber-filled), which both nourish those gut bugs and have numerous vitamins and minerals that support our health. Branch out and try some new ones like millet, buckwheat, and amaranth.

FOODS TO EAT IN MODERATION

The following are all foods that are okay in moderate amounts. You can continue to enjoy these, just a little less frequently.

Coffee and Red Wine: Coffee and red wine consumption can be beneficial to overall health, and specifically to the bacteria in our guts, because of their high polyphenol content. But the reason I did not put these two elixirs in the "Foods to Eat Freely" list is because I want to emphasize the importance of drinking alcohol mindfully and to acknowledge that copious amounts of coffee may also turn some individuals into a whirling dervish. So, enjoy your coffee and wine in moderation.

*Dairy: Some tolerate this food group much better than others, but for those for who deal with lactose intolerance, it's best to be mindful about the amount and type you are consuming. Fermented or cultured dairy like kefir or yogurt are your best bets, as the bacteria included in them naturally break down, or eat, the lactose that can cause issues. Additionally, many dairy products, such as ice cream and cheese, are usually high in fat, which can have a less favorable impact on bacterial life when consumed in large amounts.

Emulsifiers and Food Additives like Gums, Carrageenan, and Maltodextrin: Members of the gum family like guar gum, gellan gum, xanthan gum, and carrageenan are often not well digested by certain individuals, so be sure you are mindful about how much of these gums you're consuming daily and whether you can correlate eating them with any symptoms. Maltodextrin, produced from vegetable starch, sounds like it should be a good thing, but it's very processed and has been linked to gut dysbiosis and inflammation in the intestinal tract. Because of individual variability, it may not be totally clear what the appropriate amount may be for each person, so moderation is a good rule to live by.

Meat: A higher intake of meat has been associated with a less diverse microbiota. While a good source of protein, animal products don't do much to feed your microbiota because they are lacking in fiber. Additionally, because of its higher content of choline and carnitine, meat may also increase the levels of TMAO in your body, which may increase your risk of heart disease. Consumers of the typical American diet tend to pile on the animal protein, and if this makes up a large portion of our meals, it usually means that it's displacing other nutrients necessary for a healthy microbiome. There is also a big difference in the quality and nutrient makeup of meat depending on the diet of the animal. For instance, beef from a cow that was fed organic meal or was pasture-raised will likely be higher in anti-inflammatory omega-3 fatty acids and protective beta-carotene. If you are someone who relies on animal protein as a way to feel satiated or connected with your culture, see if you can shoot for a higher quality. It may be more expensive, but if you eat a little less, it may all wind up being equal.

FOODS TO RESTRICT OR AVOID

I'm not a huge fan of telling people to restrict or avoid anything because this command often has the same outcome as telling a kid, "Don't touch," and waiting to see what happens. It flares the desire to do just that.

Restriction can equal deprivation in the minds of many, which can backfire and lead to overeating some of the very items that you're working to avoid. That being said, you may find that when you focus on eating minimal amounts of the following foods, you just feel better—and that can provide more incentive to cut them out than any I can give.

Cured and Processed Meat: While some methods of curing meat may actually have benefits associated with fermented foods, sandwich meats and cured items like bacon have also been associated with higher levels of the families of bad bacteria. Additionally, high amounts of these foods in the diet is linked to a higher risk of heart disease, colon cancer, and overall inflammation. So, make bacon an infrequent treat.

Excessive Alcohol: Excessive intake of hard alcohol, hard cider, and beer can be damaging to our good bacteria, which may lead to an environment that invites potential disease. If you're struggling with a lot of digestive or inflammatory issues, your body might do well with a break from alcohol, even for a short period of time.

Excessive Simple Sugars: Most people won't argue that sugary foods and excessive refined carbohydrates don't have much to offer human health in general. They provide calories with minimal nutritional value and, in large amounts, can contribute to numerous inflammatory conditions. As previously mentioned, our more maleficent microbes also thrive on this food group, so the less we have of it, the more insurance we have that these bad bugs won't dominate our intestinal tract. These foods include sweets made with actual sugar but also include sweet and savory foodstuffs made with white processed flour, which breaks down quite rapidly into simple sugars in our body. It also includes fructose or high-fructose corn syrup found in numerous processed foods and beverages, which, according to a study published by BioMed Central, have specifically been shown to alter beneficial short-chain fatty acids and damage the intestinal wall.

FOODS TO ENJOY AND AVOID

FOODS TO ENJOY FREELY	FOODS TO EAT IN MODERATION	FOODS TO RESTRICT OR AVOID
• Alliums: Onions, Leeks, Garlic, and Scallions • Beans, Legumes, and Pulses • Brightly Colored Fruits and Vegetables • Herbs and Spices • Nuts, Seeds, and Their Respective Butters • Starchy Vegetables • Teas • Unprocessed Whole Grains	• Coffee and Red Wine • Dairy • Emulsifiers and Food Additives Like Gums, Carrageenan, and Maltodextrin • Meat	• Cured and Processed Meats • Excessive Alcohol • Excessive Simple Sugars, Refined Carbohydrates, and High-Fructose Corn Syrup

WHAT ABOUT FASTING?

When you eat and how long you wait between meals could also make a difference to your microbial health. Some preliminary research is showing that a practice called prolonged nightly fasting—a type of intermittent fasting—may improve gut barrier function, reduce inflammation, and increase our bacterial diversity. This practice promotes the consumption of all meals in a shorter window of time during the day. Essentially, this means having a 12-to-16-hour period between your last meal of the day and the next meal the following day. For example, this could mean finishing dinner at 6 p.m. on Tuesday and not having your next meal until 8 or 9 a.m. the following morning. This may sound difficult, but it's certainly worth a try. Many of my clients adopted this practice, even just a few times a week, and it has improved their sleep, aided digestive function, and helped with weight loss. If you are prone to low blood sugar or are a night owl, you may need to make modifications. It's a good idea to check with your doctor about this, as well.

WHAT ABOUT PERSONALIZED NUTRITION?

It's essential to acknowledge that these are general guidelines and don't necessarily apply to all people. If you and I were sitting across from each other in person, the recommendations might shift slightly—FODMAP avoiders may not be the only ones who need to be mindful of indiscriminately eating all the foods mentioned here. Current digestive issues or history of inflammatory bowel issues and ethnic background can also make a difference in terms of tolerance. For instance, many individuals of Asian, African, and Latino descent tend to be less tolerant of dairy due to the lack of the enzyme lactase, which can reduce tolerance to lactose, the sugar found in dairy. Fortunately, most of the dairy products discussed in the diet section are fermented or cultured, meaning they contain a lower lactose content because that milk "sugar" has been consumed and fermented by the bacteria in it. People who have lived with ulcerative colitis, Crohn's disease, or other digestive impairments may also find that dairy and/or certain beans, grains, or raw vegetables don't sit well with them.

This isn't the case across the board, and I certainly am not able to predict how everyone will respond to each food group suggested. It can be helpful to keep a food journal for this. You know your body best. It's up to you to tune into any changes you may experience when you eat these foods (pleasant or unpleasant) and to make modifications accordingly.

The Microbiome-Friendly Shopper's Guide

The market has recently exploded with products that claim to be good for you, whether they're probiotics that have more than 10 billion strains or personal care products that are free of sulfates, parabens, and other dizzying terms. What should you be prioritizing? Let's take a look.

DO I NEED SUPPLEMENTS?

This is not meant to be a comprehensive guide to supplements, which could be its own book. Instead, these are some ideas to get you started, especially if you're in the dark about these little nuggets of life in a bottle.

When it comes to supplements, I fall somewhere between enthusiast and healthy skeptic. This mostly comes back to the ever-present and forever-applicable fact that people are different. I do believe that certain people with long-standing health issues need extra support, but that doesn't mean that every supplement will work for everyone with the same symptoms. It's also about quality control. The supplemental industry is largely unregulated, so there are hundreds of supplements out there making all kinds of claims, many of which are unsubstantiated, including whether the "live" organisms in the bottle are, in fact, still alive. Bacteria like to hang out in very stable environments, so as soon as they are exposed to oxygen and heat for lengthy periods of time, they can either die off or become less effective.

That being said, numerous studies on probiotic supplemental interventions have demonstrated positive effects on the gut by increasing the production of short-chain fatty acids and helping restore balance to a disrupted microbial community. Supplemental probiotic interventions have shown beneficial results, including improved digestion, decreased rheumatoid arthritis conditions, improved cognitive symptoms associated with neurological issues such as Alzheimer's disease and Parkinson's disease, and a reduction in anxiety and depression. Many studies are small. Many are short term. Many are done on animals—and, really, how does one objectively determine that a mouse no longer has the blues? This doesn't mean these studies aren't worth paying attention to, but it means that we cannot always hang our hat on the results. The challenge around effective recommendations often has much to do with a lack of consistent results that point specifically to which strain to consume, how much to consume, and who will benefit.

Probiotics are essentially live microorganisms that offer a benefit to the host when given in sufficient quantities. Most common supplements include the lactic-acid-producing strains Bifidobacterium (often low in those with IBS) and Lactobacillus. When it comes to these two families of organisms, there is very strong research to support probiotic supplemental administration as a therapy for those with inflammatory bowel issues like ulcerative colitis, especially resulting from the pathogenic bacteria C. diff, which often arises from frequent antibiotic usage. In terms of other applications, some research around the specific strains B. Longum and L. Helveticus indicates helpfulness for depression and anxiety, and a recent study showed that supplementation with a species called Akkermansia muciniphila helped regulate appetite.

Additionally, the very well-studied probiotic yeast called Saccharomyces boulardii has been shown to have multiple beneficial effects on the altered microbiota, helping prevent and treat antibiotic-associated diarrhea. It's also helpful when it comes to preserving and restoring intestinal barrier function. If you are currently taking or have taken numerous courses of antibiotics, I strongly suggest that you consider seeking out a supplement that includes this particular yeast strain. Be sure to always take your probiotics at a different time from your antibiotic, or you run the risk of a major mob hit on the good guys.

You can also supplement with prebiotics. Not to be confused with probiotics (the stuff found in yogurt), prebiotics are compounds that provide sustenance to the probiotics or good bacteria that we either ingest or already have living in our gut. In fact, numerous probiotic supplements, termed "symbiotics," come with their own built-in prebiotic fiber source (usually inulin and fructo-oligosaccharides, or FOS) to help promote bacterial growth. However, numerous studies in both animals and humans showed great benefit to the host from consuming prebiotics only. Beneficial bacteria thrived, blood markers of cardiovascular health improved, body fat decreased, and inflammatory issues like joint pain subsided.

Of course, if you have more thriving bacteria in your gut to begin with, results may be different from someone whose biota has seen better days.

Because of the connection between the gut microbiome and inflammation, it's also reasonable to theorize that anti-inflammatory compounds may be supportive. Research around supplementing with omega-3 fatty acids, found in fish and algae oils, is still emerging, but this may also be a worthwhile experiment for improving gut health and addressing inflammation. In general, a higher intake of omega-3s is correlated with a greater diversity of gut bugs. This means that food sources of these fatty acids are going to be your friends—bring on the walnuts, chia and flax, and (if you're open to eating seafood) fatty fish.

In my professional experience, I have seen many patients improve with probiotic supplementation, whether it has made them feel fuller and more balanced, cleared up GI systems, or helped them get through winter without a cold. I've also had distressed patients call me to say, "Help! I've got gas!" after taking supplements. Then there have been patients for whom nothing has occurred with additional supplementation, but most of those folks had very few digestive issues at baseline. In most cases, however, I will tell you that there has been benefit, which leads me to believe that if you have the funds, it's worth an experiment—even if only for a month to see how you fare.

If you have been experiencing extremely compromised gut health, you might do well with a simple, short-term support-and-repair protocol. Taking digestive enzymes with meals may give your digestive fire a boost and adding zinc picolinate (25mg/day) can help repair cellular damage. Finally, some research indicates that supplemental glutamine may help protect the gut from atrophy or injury and can also nourish the gut wall, assist in intestinal repair, and maintain overall gut integrity and digestion.

You may also want to consider purchasing more natural household cleaning and personal care products to avoid the continued demise of the good bacteria in and on your body. Many of the current antibacterial brands out there are likely to be filled with potentially harmful chemicals that may not serve your bacterial community or your overall health.

WHAT TO LOOK FOR

In terms of supplements, if it's cheap, it probably doesn't have a lot of value. You get what you pay for when it comes to probiotics, so a high-quality product is not going to be $2.99 for a 60-pill bottle. It may run you closer to $29.

Unless you know you have a specific condition and have been told by a medical practitioner to seek out certain species to address a particular issue, it can be helpful to have a broad spectrum of species within a probiotic, as it casts a wider net. However, you may want to start slowly. Some brands have 80 billion (that's right, *billion*) organisms in there, although there may only be 5 to 10 species contained. That is a heck of a lot of critters to introduce, so I tend to suggest that folks start off with 10 billion organisms—or 5 billion if you are super sensitive—and build up gradually. Also, you may want to start this process in a well-ventilated room by yourself with some natural air freshener nearby.

Please remember that the efficacy of these strains may have to do with a person's baseline microbial profile, and in some cases, understanding one's initial bacterial pattern can help predict the success of the intervention.

Here is just a handful of examples of brands that have been well studied and/or contain multi-strain formulations.

Probiotics

- Align Probiotic
- Innate Response Formulas Flora 50-14
- Jarrow Formulas Jarro-Dophilus
- Klaire Labs Ther-Biotic Complete
- Microbiome Labs MegaSporeBiotic
- Visbiome (formerly VSL)

The following are examples of products containing prebiotics. This is just a smattering of the brands that I trust and that have some research to back up their claims.

Prebiotics

- BiomeBliss Powder (contains beta-glucans, polyphenols, and prebiotics)
- Jarrow Formulas Inulin-FOS
- Klaire Labs Biotagen
- Microbiome Labs MegaPre
- NOW's Prebiotic Bifido Boost Powder
- Pure Encapsulations Poly-Prebiotic powder (contains polyphenols and prebiotics)

There are also some natural brands for your personal care (things you slather on your body, including underarms, face, and hair) that are less likely to destroy the good gut bacteria. This includes toothpaste and mouthwash, which, although we do our best not to swallow them, may make their way down into our stomachs in small amounts and kill off helpful bacteria.

In general, seek out products that are organic or use essential oils in their formulations. Avoid chlorinated and fluoridated items if possible. Unfortunately, the word "natural" has very little meaning these days, so don't bet on it as an accurate descriptor—although it's less probable that a highly chemicalized product will tout itself as natural. A bonus of using these products is that they are all a bit kinder to our environment, which is in dire need of extra care these days.

Hair and Body Care

- Acure
- Avalon Organics
- Beautycounter
- Jason Organic

Household Cleaners

- Biokleen
- Ecover
- Method
- Seventh Generation

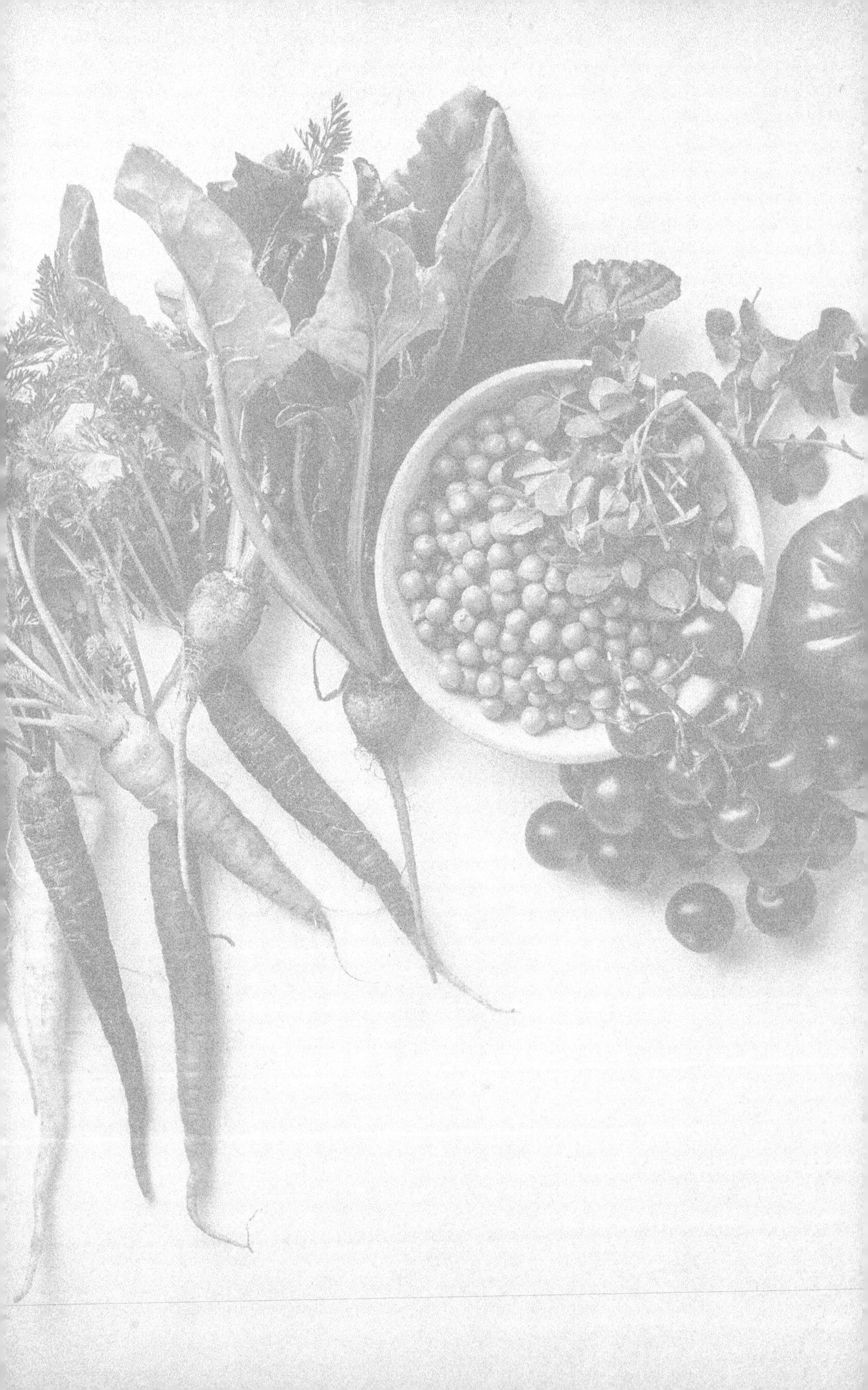

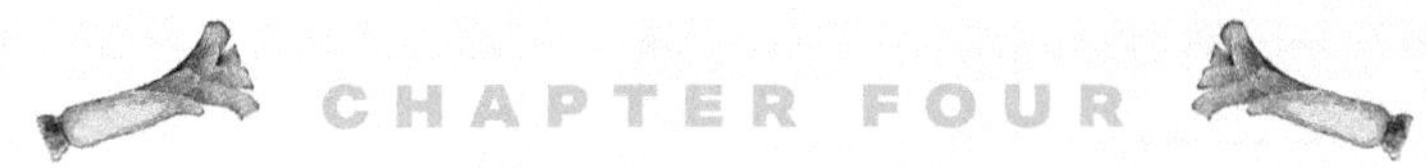

The Microbiome Diet Meal Plan

Maybe you've been cooking your own meals since you were in high school. Or perhaps you've lived at deli counters, drive-thrus, and diners for the past decade. No matter your experience in the kitchen, it can be helpful to have a bit of structure as you embark on this GI journey. As someone who rarely follows a plan to the letter, I welcome you to think of these meal plans as flexible blueprints and suggestions of what a week of microbiome-supportive eating might look like. You can mix and match as you see fit. There's no need to have a black bean salad for lunch on a Thursday if you are in the mood for lentil curry. Don't like cilantro? Swap it out for parsley. The idea is to eat these *kinds* of foods. Beyond that, feel free to tailor it to your individual likes and dislikes.

Realistic Meal Planning

Remember how great it was to start a school essay with an outline already in hand? Meal plans can be a little like that. Instead of the obligation to read and synthesize the information you've ingested and magically put all the pieces together on your own, some of that guesswork and preparation has been taken off your hands. When you don't have to come up with ideas for the eating strategies, it's a lot easier to execute the plan.

Whatever your personal weekend is, this is a great time to shop, plan, and do a little bit of cooking so that you can start day 1 (Monday or not) with some ready-to-eat (or at least chopped and ready-to-cook) food in the refrigerator that you can bring with you or leave waiting for you upon your return from the day's events.

I've formulated the plan for you so that:

1. You aren't cooking three full meals each day that you don't have time for. There's always an easily assembled meal included daily.
2. You've got both hot and cold dish options during the day, depending on what your personal preference may be. (Sometimes it's just too darn chilly for a salad or just too hot for a spicy stew.)
3. There's enough repetition of ingredients so that you may not have to cook and chop as much over the course of a few days, but not so much repetition that you wind up with chard or cilantro three times in one day.
4. You have leftovers. I've suggested doubling up on breakfast and transforming some of the dinners into leftovers for lunch to reduce your time in the kitchen. If you aren't a leftover lover, feel free to revise and add your own personal organizational flair.

Finally, I've thrown in a few thought-free snack ideas because you may need some nosh in the late afternoon! You're welcome to choose similar versions of these simple items. When in doubt, fruit and nuts always make a perfect no-brainer, grab-and-go boost.

Be sure to also take a look at the recipes in chapter 5 and chapter 6 for some targeted dishes that are specifically rich in prebiotics and probiotics. Some of these items may also be perfect for snacks or side dishes with a probiotic punch.

Weekly Meal Plans with Shopping Lists

The following takes you through a seven-day meal plan with a shopping list that includes all the necessary ingredients. If you have a favorite go-to meal of your own, feel free to throw it into the mix. I promise that the other recipes won't mind.

REGULAR MEAL PLAN

	SNACKS	BREAKFAST	LUNCH	DINNER
MON	Handful of nuts or seeds (10 walnuts or ¼ cup sunflower seeds)	Buckwheat Bliss Bowl (page 66)	Kale Salad with White Beans and Jicama (page 72)	Four-Bean Chili (page 78)
TUE	A hardboiled egg and piece of fruit	Banana Berry Kefir Smoothie (page 64)	Leftover Four-Bean Chili	One-Pot Chicken with Jerusalem Artichokes and Potatoes (page 88)
WED	Yogurt or kefir with fruit and a drizzle of maple syrup	Asparagus and Leek Omelet with Garlic Roasted Potatoes (page 68)	Leftover One-Pot Chicken with Jerusalem Artichokes and Potatoes	Lentil Curry with Sweet Potatoes and Raita (page 82)
THU	Raw vegetables with almond butter	Overnight Chia Pudding (page 65)	Leftover Lentil Curry with Sweet Potatoes and Raita	Mediterranean Quinoa Salad (page 83)
FRI	Hummus with vegetables	Banana Berry Kefir Smoothie (page 64)	Red Passion Hummus Vegetable Sandwich (page 74)	Thai Fish Stew (page 86)

continued›

	SNACKS	BREAKFAST	LUNCH	DINNER
SAT	Handful of nuts or seeds (15 cashews or ¼ cup pumpkin seeds)	Leftover Overnight Chia Pudding	Black Bean Salad (page 75)	Eggplant, Tofu, and Edamame Stir-Fry (page 80)
SUN	Veggies with sunflower seed butter	Green Shakshuka (page 67)	Tempeh Reuben Sandwich (page 70)	Miso-Tamari Soba Noodles with Chicken (page 89)

Shopping List

VEGETABLES

Artichokes, Jerusalem (8 ounces)

Asparagus (6, or 1 bunch)

Beet (1)

Bell pepper, red (1)

Carrots, medium (3)

Corn (1 bag frozen or 3 fresh)

Cucumbers (3)

Green beans (½ pound)

Eggplant, Japanese (1 pound)

Jicama, small (1)

Kale (1 bunch)

Mushrooms, white (5)

Potato, sweet (1)

Potatoes, red or purple, medium (3)

Potatoes, red, small (2 to 3, or 8 ounces)

Radishes (2 bunches)

Sauerkraut, unpasteurized (1 jar)

Spinach (1 bunch)

Sprouts, alfalfa or sunflower (1 container)

Vegetables, of choice (3 servings)

Zucchini, medium (1)

FRUITS

Avocados (2)

Bananas (2)

Berries, of choice (2 pints)

Dates or figs, dried (¼ cup)

Fruit, of choice (2 servings)

Lemons (4)

Limes (5)

Tomatoes, Roma (7)

HERBS, SPICES, AND ALLIUMS

- Basil, dried
- Cardamom, ground
- Cilantro, fresh (1 bunch)
- Cinnamon, ground
- Cumin, ground
- Curry powder
- Garlic (2 bulbs)
- Garlic powder
- Ginger root, 1 (1-inch) piece
- Leek (1)
- Mustard seeds
- Onion powder
- Onion, red (1)
- Onion, yellow (3)
- Oregano, dried
- Paprika
- Parsley, fresh (1 bunch)
- Pepper, black
- Rosemary, fresh (2 sprigs)
- Salt, sea
- Scallions (9, or 1 bunch)
- Thyme, fresh (1 small bunch)
- Turmeric, ground

GRAINS

- Bread, gluten-free, sprouted whole-wheat, or sourdough (1 loaf)
- Buckwheat groats (1 cup)
- Lentils, brown (1 cup, available in bulk sections)
- Quinoa (3 cups)

PROTEIN SOURCES AND YOGURTS/KEFIRS

- Chicken, boneless, skinless breasts (2 pounds)
- Chicken, bone-in thighs (4)
- Edamame, frozen shelled (1 bag)
- Eggs (1 dozen)
- Hummus (1 package)
- Kefir, plain (6 cups)
- Tempeh, 1 (8-ounce) package
- Tofu, firm, 1 (8-ounce) package
- Whitefish fillets (12 ounces)
- Yogurt, coconut milk, 1 (16-ounce) container
- Yogurt or kefir, of choice (1 serving)

NUTS AND SEEDS

Butter, almond

Butter, sunflower seed

Cashews (¼ cup)

Flaxseed, ground (½ cup)

Seeds, chia (½ cup)

Seeds, sesame (½ cup)

Seeds, sunflower (¼ cup)

Walnuts (½ cup)

BOXED/CANNED GOODS

Beans, black, 3 (15-ounce) cans

Beans, kidney, 1 (15-ounce) can

Beans, pinto, 1 (15-ounce) can

Beans, white, 1 (15-ounce) can

Broth, chicken or bone, 1 (8-ounce) carton

Broth, vegetable or bone, 2 (32-ounce) cartons

Chickpeas, 2 (15-ounce) cans

Lentils, 1 (15-ounce) can

Milk, coconut, full-fat, 2 (13.5-ounce) cans

Noodles, buckwheat soba, 1 (8-ounce) package

Peppers, chipotle in adobo, 1 can

Tomato paste, 1 (6-ounce) can

CONDIMENTS

Curry paste, Thai red

Fish sauce

Honey

Horseradish

Miso paste

Oil, extra-virgin olive

Oil, sesame, toasted

Sugar, coconut

Syrup, maple

Tahini

Tamari

Vinegar, rice wine

Sensitive System Meal Plan

As promised, there is a plan for those with sensitive stomachs. There will be fewer items from both the FODMAPs family and fermented foods section in this version. Keep in mind that, depending on what your gut health baseline is, it may be necessary to follow this plan for a longer period of time than just one week in order to see improvement.

SENSITIVE SYSTEM MEAL PLAN

	SNACKS	BREAKFAST	LUNCH	DINNER
MON	A hardboiled egg and piece of fruit	Buckwheat Bliss Bowl (page 66)	Kale Salad with White Beans and Jicama (replace beans with your favorite protein source) page 72)	One-Pot Chicken with Jerusalem Artichokes and Potatoes (page 88)
TUE	Handful of nuts or seeds (10 walnuts or ¼ cup sunflower seeds)	Banana Berry Kefir Smoothie (page 64)	Leftover One-Pot Chicken with Jerusalem Artichokes and Potatoes	Whitefish in Parchment with Vegetables (page 84)
WED	Carrots with tahini (sesame seed butter)	Asparagus and Leek Omelet (replace asparagus with zucchini) (page 68)	Leftover Whitefish in Parchment with Vegetables	Mediterranean Quinoa Salad (page 83)
THU	Handful of nuts or seeds (10 walnuts or ¼ cup sunflower seeds)	Oatmeal with nuts, seeds, and berries and your choice of milk	Leftover Zucchini and Leek Omelet	Salmon Burger Wrap with Sweet Potato Fries (page 76)

continued ›

	SNACKS	BREAKFAST	LUNCH	DINNER
FRI	Coconut milk yogurt/kefir with fruit and a drizzle of maple syrup	Banana Berry Kefir Smoothie (page 64)	Leftover Mediterranean Quinoa Salad	Miso-Tamari Soba Noodles with Chicken (page 89)
SAT	A hardboiled egg and piece of fruit	Buckwheat Bliss Bowl (page 66)	Leftover Miso-Tamari Soba Noodles with Chicken	Thai Fish Stew (page 86)
SUN	Handful of nuts or seeds (10 walnuts or ¼ cup pumpkin seeds)	Green Shakshuka (page 67)	Leftover Thai Fish Stew	Eggplant, Tofu, and Edamame Stir-Fry (replace tofu with chicken) (page 80)

Shopping List

VEGETABLES

Artichoke, Jerusalem (8 ounces)

Bell peppers, red (2)

Bok choy, large head (1)

Carrots, medium (3)

Cucumber (1)

Eggplant, Japanese (1 pound)

Green beans (1 pound)

Jicama, small (1)

Kale (1 bunch)

Lettuce, small head (1)

Mushrooms, white, 1 small package

Potatoes, red, medium (3)

Potatoes, red or purple, small (8 ounces)

Potatoes, sweet, medium (4)

Spinach (1 bunch)

Zucchini, medium (4)

FRUITS

Avocado (1)

Bananas (2)

Berries, of choice (3 pints)

Fruit, of choice (3 servings)

Lemons (4)

Limes (4)

Tomatoes, Roma (2)

HERBS, SPICES, AND ALLIUMS

Basil, dried

Cilantro, fresh (1 bunch)

Cinnamon, ground

Cumin, ground

Garlic, 1 bulb

Garlic powder

Ginger root, 1 (4-inch) piece

Leek (1)

Onions, yellow (1)

Oregano, dried

Parsley, fresh (1 bunch)

Pepper, black

Red pepper flakes

Rosemary, fresh (2 sprigs)

Salt, sea

Scallions (15)

Scallions, chopped (½ cup)

Thyme, fresh (1 small bunch)

GRAINS

Buckwheat groats (2 cups)

Oatmeal (1 serving)

Quinoa (1 cup)

PROTEIN SOURCES AND YOGURTS/KEFIRS

Chicken, bone-in thighs (4)

Chicken, boneless, skinless breasts (2 pounds)

Chicken, of choice (8 ounces)

Edamame, shelled, frozen (1 bag)

Egg (1 dozen)

Kefir, plain (4 cups)

Protein, of choice (15 ounces)

Whitefish, fillets (3 pounds)

Yogurt, coconut milk, 1 (32-ounce) container

NUTS AND SEEDS

Flaxseed (½ cup)

Nuts, of choice (1 serving)

Seeds, of choice (1 serving)

Seeds, pumpkin (¼ cup)

Seeds, sesame (½ cup)

Seeds, sunflower (¾ cup)

Walnuts (1 cup)

BOXED/CANNED GOODS

Broth, chicken or bone, 1 (8-ounce) carton

Broth, vegetable or bone, 1 (32-ounce) carton

Chickpeas, 1 (15-ounce) can

Flour, arrowroot (3 tablespoons)

Milk, coconut, full-fat, 1 (13.5-ounce) can

Milk, of choice (1 serving)

Noodles, buckwheat soba, 1 (8-ounce) package

Salmon, boneless, skinless, 2 (6-ounce) cans

CONDIMENTS

Curry paste, Thai red

Fish sauce

Honey

Miso paste

Oil, extra-virgin olive

Oil, toasted sesame

Sugar, coconut

Syrup, maple

Tahini

Tamari

Vinegar, rice wine

Effort-Saving Tips and Tricks

Here are five ways to speed up your meal preparation so that you have more time to do the things you love with all that newfound energy.

1. **Organize and clean your kitchen.** There's nothing that keeps us out of the kitchen more than dirty dishes in the sink, clutter on the counter, and a refrigerator that contains unrecognizable items. Give yourself an hour (or more) to clean this area so that your food prep experience isn't overwhelming. Do you know where that favorite spatula, soup bowl, or cast-iron pan is amid the cookware in your cabinets? Locate them and keep them accessible so that you can grab them without a hunt.
2. **Batch cook.** Cook once and eat thrice! Unless you tire very easily of certain foods or fear your freezer, it can be wonderful to make a large batch of whatever you are cooking so that you have leftovers either for the next day or the week.

3. **Wash and chop up a bunch of your vegetables so that they are there and ready to go.** Have you ever said, "But I don't feel like chopping vegetables"? This is one of the biggest deterrents to eating vegetables, so why not make it happen in one standing (preferably as you are unpacking your groceries)? Get out your knife, your cutting board, and some handy glass Tupperware to store those chopped vegetables (or place them in a plastic bag in the freezer). The next time you open your refrigerator, you'll have ready-to-go vegetables for your salad, soup, stew, or dip.
4. **Bring those kitchen gadgets into sight.** These can be simple items, like the cutting board, a peeler, or a zester, or bigger ticket items, like the blender, food processor, or slow cooker. These gadgets were created to make your life easier. If you see them, you're more likely to use them.
5. **Utilize precooked/prepared foods.** You may not have time to soak beans, make vegetable broth, or ferment your own cabbage. Luckily, there are food companies in this world that have made it their mission to do just that for you. You are no less of a good person if you use canned beans, boxed vegetable broth, or chopped or jarred vegetables. Sometimes a helping hand is just the thing that gets you over the hurdle of what might be a daunting task. It may even help you love the process of cooking (or meal assembling) even more.

About the Recipes

When it comes to the recipes in this book, there is a little something for everyone. Whether it's about time, ease, simplicity, or sensitivity, we've got you covered. In the big picture, all the recipes focus on vibrant, unprocessed, and fiber-packed meals that are meant to give your good bacteria the feast of a lifetime. There is no refined sugar or red or processed meat, and there is very little dairy—except the fermented or cultured kind. The bread I suggest buying is sprouted, sourdough, or rye, all of which can be easier to digest.

There are also recipes provided here that are specifically indicated for people who are either following, or thinking of experimenting with, a low-FODMAPs diet, who may have trouble digesting certain foods. I have labeled these recipes as such. In general, anytime you see the high-FODMAP ingredients garlic or onions, feel free to utilize the Onion-and-Garlic-Infused Oil recipe (see page 61), or try making it with scallions or the spice asafetida, which has a great flavor combination of garlic and onions with a hint of celery. Gluten-free or 100 percent rye bread will be the best option for sandwiches.

To keep things easy, all recipes will fall under one of the following categories and will be labeled as such:

5-Ingredient: These require five main ingredients, not including oil, water, salt, or pepper.

One-Pot: These dishes can be cooked using a single pot or bowl.

One-Pan: These dishes can be made in a single skillet or sheet pan.

30-Minute: These dishes can be prepped, cooked, and served in 30 minutes or less.

Low-FODMAP: These dishes conform to the low-FODMAP diet.

BAM! Dinner is on the table.

ONION-AND-GARLIC-INFUSED OIL

½ cup extra-virgin olive oil

1 yellow onion, quartered

3 garlic cloves, crushed

1. In a small pot, combine the oil, onion, and garlic and cook over low heat until the garlic and onion begin simmering. Remove the pot from the heat and let the oil cool to room temperature, about 1 hour.
2. Using a strainer, remove the onion and garlic pieces and discard. Transfer the oil to an airtight container and store in the refrigerator for 3 to 4 days.

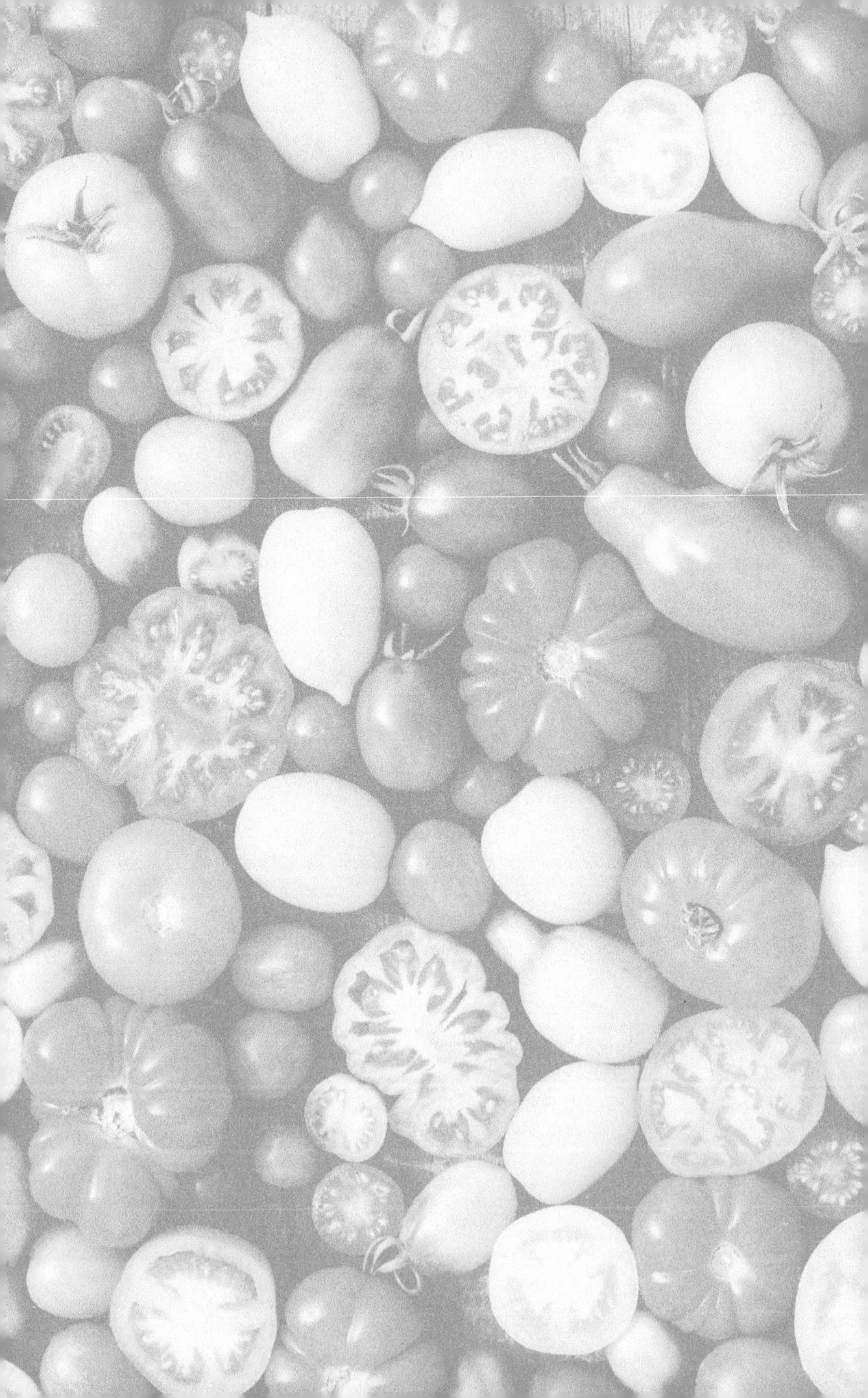

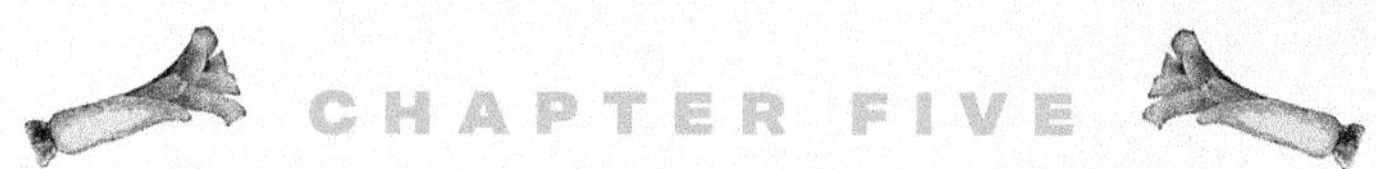

CHAPTER FIVE

Recipes for Prebiotic-Packed Meals

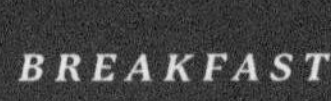

Banana Berry Kefir Smoothie

30-MINUTE, 5-INGREDIENT

SERVES 2

PREP TIME 5 minutes

Similar to a thin yogurt, kefir is a fermented milk drink that is loaded with probiotic bacteria for a healthy gut. Flaxseed is a good source of fiber, protein, and alpha-linolenic acid (ALA), an essential omega-3 fatty acid, making them a perfect addition to any breakfast smoothie to get you going in the morning. Combined with the sweetness from berries and banana, this smoothie is perfect for regular use in your meal rotation.

2 cups plain kefir

1 banana, frozen

½ cup blueberries, raspberries, or strawberries

¼ cup ground flaxseed

Juice of 1 lime

Ice

In a blender, combine the kefir, banana, berries, flaxseed, and lime juice. Blend until smooth. Add 2 to 3 ice cubes (or more for a thicker consistency) and blend until smooth.

Variation tip: To make this dairy-free, opt for a plant-based kefir, like one made with coconut milk.

FODMAP-Friendly tip: Use a less ripe banana or substitute a small slice of avocado for the banana instead.

Per serving: Calories: 299, Total fat: 11g; Saturated fat: 4g; Protein: 13g; Carbohydrates: 41g; Fiber: 6g; Sodium: 124mg

Overnight Chia Pudding

ONE-POT

SERVES 4

PREP TIME 5 minutes, plus 2 hours to chill

Chia seeds become thick and wonderfully sticky when soaked in liquid, making them a great base for a healthy breakfast pudding loaded with omega-3s. Sticky and sweet with concentrated natural sugars, dates are a good source of fiber, iron, and potassium. Swap them with other seasonal berries and chopped stone fruits as available to make this pudding an easy breakfast year-round. If you prefer a smooth pudding, blend the ingredients in step 1 before refrigerating.

- 2 cups plain kefir
- ½ cup chia seeds
- ½ teaspoon ground cardamom
- ¼ cup chopped dried dates or figs
- ¼ cup walnut pieces
- 4 teaspoons honey

1. In a medium bowl, stir together the kefir, chia seeds, and cardamom. Cover and refrigerate for about 2 hours, stirring once or twice, until set and chilled.
2. To serve, divide into bowls and evenly top with the dates, walnuts, and honey.

Preparation tip: Chia pudding is great for meal prepping. Divide the recipe into separate single serving jars and top with fruit and walnuts before serving. Chia pudding can be refrigerated in an airtight container for up to five days.

FODMAP-Friendly tip: Substitute your favorite fresh berries for the dried fruit and use maple syrup in place of honey.

Per serving: Calories: 297; Total fat: 14g; Saturated fat: 2g; Protein: 12g; Carbohydrates: 34g; Fiber: 12g; Sodium: 61mg

Buckwheat Bliss Bowl

30-MINUTE, 5-INGREDIENT, LOW-FODMAP

SERVES	PREP TIME	COOK TIME
4	5 minutes	20 minutes

While its name may imply otherwise, buckwheat is not part of the wheat family—it's actually a gluten-free, grain-like seed. Buckwheat is rich in fiber, and the antioxidants rutin and catechin, earning it a reputation as a superfood. This ancient grain is cultivated around the world and used in many applications, including pancakes, breads, and noodles. Here it's combined with yogurt and fresh fruit for a delightful breakfast bowl.

- 2 cups water
- 1 cup buckwheat groats, rinsed
- 2 cups berries (blueberries, raspberries, strawberries)
- 2 cups coconut milk yogurt
- ¼ cup walnut halves or hemp seeds
- ½ teaspoon ground cinnamon

1. In a small pot, combine the water and buckwheat and bring to a boil over medium-high heat. Cover the pot, reduce the heat to low, and simmer for 10 minutes, then turn off the heat and let rest for 5 minutes, covered.
2. Fluff the buckwheat with a fork and transfer to serving bowls. Top with the berries, yogurt, walnuts, and cinnamon and serve.

Ingredient tip: Cooked buckwheat can be stored in an airtight container in the refrigerator for up to a week, making it perfect for meal prepping. Use it in place of rice and quinoa. When using it in the morning from leftovers, you can heat the cold buckwheat in the microwave before topping and serving.

Per serving: Calories: 319; Total fat: 10g; Saturated fat: 4g; Protein: 8g; Carbohydrates: 54g; Fiber: 10g; Sodium: 11mg

Green Shakshuka

30-MINUTE, ONE-POT

SERVES	PREP TIME	COOK TIME
2	15 minutes	15 minutes

Shakshuka is a traditional Israeli and North African breakfast food made of simmered spiced tomatoes with poached eggs. Here it gets a green makeover in this flavorful blend featuring spinach and zucchini. Spinach is supportive of the digestive tract and, because of its mild taste, is easy to incorporate into your diet. If you need a little more food in the morning, enjoy this with a slice of toasted sprouted wheat or sourdough bread.

- 1 tablespoon extra-virgin olive oil
- 1 small yellow onion, finely chopped
- 1 medium zucchini, grated
- 4 cups packed thinly sliced spinach
- 3 scallions, white and green parts, thinly sliced
- 1 teaspoon ground cumin
- Sea salt
- Freshly ground black pepper
- 4 large eggs
- ½ avocado, sliced, for serving
- 2 tablespoons chopped fresh cilantro, for serving

1. In a large skillet, heat the oil over medium-high heat and sauté the onion for 3 to 5 minutes, until softened.
2. Add the zucchini and spinach and sauté for 2 to 3 minutes, until the spinach is wilted.
3. Stir in the scallions and cumin and heat for about 1 minute. Season with salt and pepper.
4. Form four small wells in the spinach mixture and crack an egg into each well. Cover and cook for 5 to 7 minutes, depending on how you like your eggs cooked.
5. Serve the shakshuka topped with avocado slices and cilantro.

Variation tip: Use a large bunch of Swiss chard or bok choy in place of the spinach and zucchini and sauté the chopped greens and stems for five to seven minutes, until the stems are tender, before moving on with the recipe.

Per serving: Calories: 331; Total fat: 24g; Saturated fat: 5g; Protein: 18g; Carbohydrates: 15g; Fiber: 7g; Sodium: 211mg

Asparagus and Leek Omelet with Garlic Roasted Potatoes

30-MINUTE

SERVES	PREP TIME	COOK TIME
2	10 minutes	15 minutes

Asparagus, leeks, and fresh thyme work together to brighten up this breakfast classic. Put the potatoes in the oven before you start making the omelet, and you will have a complete meal ready right around the same time the omelet is done cooking. Breakfast is the perfect meal to get a jump-start on your vegetable intake for the day. If you don't like asparagus or leeks, consider using any leafy greens, scallions, mushrooms, zucchini, or broccoli instead.

- 3 medium red potatoes, cut into ½-inch dice
- 1 tablespoon extra-virgin olive oil, divided
- 6 asparagus spears, chopped
- ¼ cup thinly sliced leeks
- 4 large eggs
- 1 tablespoon minced fresh thyme leaves
- Sea salt
- Freshly ground black pepper
- 2 garlic cloves, minced

1. Preheat the oven to 400°F.
2. On a baking sheet, toss the potatoes with ½ tablespoon of oil. Spread the potatoes in a single layer and bake for 15 minutes, stirring once halfway through, until tender and lightly browned.
3. Meanwhile, in a medium skillet, heat the remaining ½ tablespoon of oil over medium-high heat. Sauté the asparagus and leek for about 5 minutes, until the leek is translucent.
4. While the vegetables are sautéing, beat the eggs in a small bowl with the thyme, then season with salt and pepper.
5. Remove the asparagus and leeks from the skillet and set aside. Pour the eggs into the skillet and reduce the heat to medium-low. Cook for 1 minute, until the bottom is set, then add the leeks and asparagus on top. Cover and cook for 2 to 3 minutes, until set.
6. When the potatoes are done, toss with the garlic, and cook for 1 more minute, until fragrant. Serve the omelet with the potatoes on the side.

Preparation tip: Prep the leek and asparagus the night before to quickly make the omelet in the morning. To speed up cooking the potatoes, you can parboil them the night before for about five minutes, until just fork-tender. Then drain, cool, and refrigerate in an airtight container. In the morning, sauté the potatoes in a skillet with the olive oil over medium-high heat until browned, then toss with the garlic.

FODMAP-Friendly tip: Use only the green portion of the leek and substitute zucchini or kale for the asparagus.

Per servings: Calories: 393; Total fat: 17g; Saturated fat: 4g; Protein: 20g; Carbohydrates: 45g; Fiber: 6g; Sodium: 146mg

Tempeh Reuben Sandwich

30-MINUTE

SERVES	PREP TIME	COOK TIME
2	10 minutes	20 minutes

This sandwich has all the great flavors of a Reuben but uses tempeh instead of the usual corned beef. Tempeh, a cooked and lightly fermented soybean product formed into a delightfully dense cake, is high in vitamins, minerals, and prebiotics. By simmering it with tamari and spices, it takes on a great umami flavor that makes this lightened-up sandwich feel meaty. It's finished with a heaped serving of sauerkraut, a microbiome superfood loaded with probiotics.

For the dressing

1 large egg yolk

Juice of ½ lemon

1 garlic clove, minced

1 cup extra-virgin olive oil

¼ cup Fermented Ketchup (page 101)

½ teaspoon prepared horseradish

For the sandwiches

2 tablespoons tamari

1 teaspoon onion powder

1 teaspoon garlic powder

½ teaspoon paprika

1 (8-ounce) package tempeh, sliced into strips

1 cup water

4 sprouted whole-wheat or sourdough bread slices, divided

1 tablespoon extra-virgin olive oil, divided

½ cup Sauerkraut (page 93) or store-bought sauerkraut (unpasteurized)

1 Roma tomato, sliced

To make the dressing

1. In a wide-mouth jar or small bowl, use an immersion blender to mix the egg yolk, lemon juice, and garlic.
2. Pour in the olive oil and blend for 2 to 4 minutes, until the oil and egg emulsify and thicken. Stir in the ketchup and horseradish and set aside.

To make the sandwiches

3. In a small pot, combine the tamari, onion powder, garlic powder, and paprika. Mix well and add the tempeh, tossing to coat. Add the water and bring to a simmer over medium heat. Cook for 10 minutes, then drain.
4. To make the sandwiches, heat a large skillet over medium-high heat. Brush 2 of the bread slices with ½ tablespoon of oil and place onto the skillet. Top each slice with a few pieces of tempeh, then add ¼ cup of sauerkraut on top. Add the tomato slices, then top with the remaining 2 pieces of bread, brushed with the remaining ½ tablespoon of oil. Cook for 3 to 4 minutes per side, flip carefully and continue to cook until golden brown. Open the side of the sandwich with the sauerkraut, top with the dressing, and serve.

Ingredient tip: Save extra dressing in an airtight container in the refrigerator for up to one week. Look for raw unpasteurized sauerkraut in the refrigerated section of the grocery store. Again, canned versions that have been pasteurized have been heated to the point of killing the beneficial bacteria that were once present.

Per serving: Calories (sandwich without dressing): 500; Total fat: 19g; Saturated fat: 3g; Protein: 31g; Carbohydrates: 54g; Fiber: 17g; Sodium: 1,407mg

Kale Salad with White Beans and Jicama

30-MINUTE

SERVES	PREP TIME
4	15 minutes

Kale salad stores well, making it a perfect recipe to have on hand for weekday lunches. The miso-sesame dressing ties the salad together with a probiotic punch, while inulin-rich beans and jicama provide prebiotic support. White beans and sunflower seeds are the protein component, but they can easily be swapped out for other beans and nuts or seeds you have on hand.

For the dressing

- 2 tablespoons rice wine vinegar
- 1 tablespoon miso paste
- 1 tablespoon extra-virgin olive oil
- 1 tablespoon toasted sesame oil
- ½ inch fresh ginger root, peeled and coarsely chopped
- 1 garlic clove, minced
- 1 teaspoon honey

For the salad

- 1 bunch kale, stemmed and thinly sliced
- Juice of ½ lemon
- 1 tablespoon extra-virgin olive oil
- 1 (15-ounce) can white beans, drained and rinsed
- ½ small jicama, peeled and thinly sliced
- ¼ cup sunflower seeds

To make the dressing

1. Combine the vinegar, miso paste, olive oil, sesame oil, ginger, garlic, and honey in a blender. Set aside.

To make the salad

2. Toss together the kale, lemon juice, and oil in a bowl. Using clean hands, massage the kale for a couple of minutes to work the oil into the leaves.
3. Toss the beans, jicama, and sunflower seeds with the kale and serve with the dressing drizzled on top.

Preparation tip: In this salad, the jicama works best when thinly shaved or sliced. I like to use a mandoline to create tiny strips, but a vegetable peeler is also a great tool for this.

FODMAP-Friendly tip: Small amounts of jicama should be tolerated, and the beans can be replaced with your favorite protein source. Go light on the honey and garlic or replace with maple syrup and your favorite herb or spice.

Per serving: Calories: 247; Total fat: 11g; Saturated fat: 2g; Protein: 8g; Carbohydrates: 31g; Fiber: 9g; Sodium: 160mg

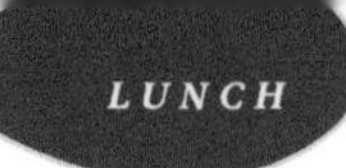

Red Passion Hummus Vegetable Sandwich

30-MINUTE

SERVES 2

PREP TIME 15 minutes

Hummus is a great way to pack in protein and fiber, but here it gets another layer of flavor and nutrition with beets. Not only do beets provide the vibrant red color of the picture-perfect sandwich, but they also are great source of fiber, folate, potassium, and vitamin C. Look for packaged roasted beets in the refrigerated section of your store's produce section.

For the hummus

1 (15-ounce) can chickpeas, drained and rinsed

1 roasted beet

¼ cup extra-virgin olive oil

2 tablespoons tahini

Juice of 1 lemon

3 garlic cloves, peeled

Sea salt

For the sandwiches

4 sprouted whole-wheat or sourdough bread slices, divided

1 cucumber, sliced

¼ cup Fermented Radishes (page 94) or other fermented vegetables

¼ cup shredded carrots

1 cup crisp sprouts (alfalfa, sunflower)

To make the hummus

1. Combine the chickpeas, beet, oil, tahini, lemon juice, and garlic in a blender. Season with salt and add a little water as needed to create a smooth, creamy consistency.

To make the sandwiches

2. Spread 3 tablespoons of the hummus each onto 2 pieces of the bread and top each with half of the cucumbers, radishes, carrots, and sprouts. Close the sandwiches with the 2 remaining pieces of bread and serve.

Per serving: Calories: 402; Total fat: 19g; Saturated fat: 3g; Protein: 16g; Carbohydrates: 49g; Fiber: 11g; Sodium: 529mg

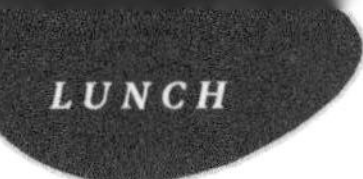

Black Bean Salad

30-MINUTE

SERVES 4

PREP TIME 10 minutes

Bean and grain salads give you a lot of bang for your buck—and your time! Once you cook your grain, this salad comes together in minutes and holds up well in the refrigerator throughout the week for an easy lunch. This plant-based salad is filling and delicious, with so much of its flavor coming from the cilantro. The phytonutrient-rich herb is anti-inflammatory and may help support healthy blood sugar levels.

- 2 (15-ounce) cans black beans, drained and rinsed
- 2 cups cooked quinoa, brown rice, or millet
- 4 Roma tomatoes, chopped
- 1 cup corn, fresh or frozen and thawed
- 1 small red onion, minced
- ½ cilantro bunch, chopped
- Juice of 2 limes
- 2 tablespoons extra-virgin olive oil
- 1 avocado, chopped
- Sea salt
- Freshly ground black pepper

1. In a large bowl, toss together the black beans, quinoa, tomatoes, corn, onion, and cilantro. Drizzle the lime juice and olive oil over the top and toss again to mix.
2. Fold in the avocado and season with salt and pepper. Serve.

Ingredient tip: To extract the most juice from the limes, roll them firmly on the counter with your palm before juicing.

FODMAP-Friendly tip: Use scallions and add grilled chicken in place of the black beans, or just halve the amount of beans in the recipe if you can tolerate that amount.

Per serving: Calories: 517; Total fat: 16g; Saturated fat: 2g; Protein: 18g; Carbohydrates: 78g; Fiber: 16g; Sodium: 20mg

Salmon Burger Wrap with Sweet Potato Fries

30-MINUTE

SERVES	PREP TIME	COOK TIME
4	5 minutes	25 minutes

Salmon burgers are an easy way to get a healthy dose of omega-3 fatty acids with very little work. By the time the burgers are done cooking, the sweet potato fries will be ready to go, and lunch is served. Pack up leftovers and store for up to three days in the refrigerator.

- 4 medium sweet potatoes, cut into thin wedges
- 2 tablespoons extra-virgin olive oil, divided
- Sea salt
- 2 (6-ounce) cans boneless, skinless salmon, drained
- 3 tablespoons arrowroot flour
- 1 large egg
- Grated zest and juice of ½ lemon
- 1 garlic clove, minced
- ¼ teaspoon red pepper flakes
- Freshly ground black pepper
- 4 large lettuce leaves, for serving

1. Preheat the oven to 400°F.
2. In a bowl, toss together the sweet potatoes and 1 tablespoon of oil. Season with salt and spread on a baking sheet in a single layer. Bake for 20 to 25 minutes or until browned, flipping once about halfway through cooking.
3. While the fries are cooking, in a bowl, combine the salmon, arrowroot flour, egg, lemon zest and juice, garlic, and red pepper flakes. Season with salt and pepper. Mix well and form into four patties. Don't worry if they are a little wet at this time—they will firm up during cooking.
4. In a large skillet, heat the remaining 1 tablespoon of oil over medium-high heat. Cook the burgers on each side for 3 to 5 minutes, flipping once, until browned and cooked through. Serve wrapped in a lettuce leaf with the fries.

Ingredient tip: Arrowroot flour, also known as arrowroot starch or arrowroot powder, is a white, powdery starch used for thickening, baking, and crisping foods. Look for it in the baking section of your grocery store, at a natural foods store, or online.

FODMAP-Friendly tip: Replace the garlic with ¼ teaspoon asafetida powder and limit sweet potatoes to ½ cup per serving.

Per serving: Calories: 338; Total fat: 10g; Saturated fat: 2g; Protein: 24g; Carbohydrates: 40g; Fiber: 4g; Sodium: 369mg

Four-Bean Chili

30-MINUTE, ONE-POT

SERVES	PREP TIME	COOK TIME
6	10 minutes	15 minutes

Beans are a powerful plant protein and prebiotic that support the growth of healthy bacteria in the gut. This chili is simple yet delicious with just a few pantry staples. Chipotle peppers in adobo is a common canned ingredient that is found in the Latin food section of the grocery store and provides the smoky flavor that is the backbone of this chili. You will have some left over in the can after making this. Refrigerate the peppers in their sauce for up to 1 month and use in other recipes to add flavor and heat.

2 tablespoons extra-virgin olive oil

1 yellow onion, chopped

4 garlic cloves, minced

2 chipotle peppers in adobo, minced

1 (15-ounce) can black beans, drained and rinsed

1 (15-ounce) can kidney beans, drained and rinsed

1 (15-ounce) can pinto beans, drained and rinsed

1 (15-ounce) can lentils, drained and rinsed

4 cups vegetable broth

2 tablespoons tomato paste

Sea salt

Freshly ground black pepper

1. In a pot, heat the oil over medium-high heat. Sauté the onion and garlic for 3 to 5 minutes, until the onion is translucent.
2. Add the chipotle peppers and cook for about 30 seconds, until fragrant.
3. Add the black beans, kidney beans, pinto beans, lentils, broth, and tomato paste and bring to a boil. Reduce the heat to simmer for 10 minutes, until thickened. Season with salt and pepper and serve.

Ingredient tip: When you use a small amount of tomato paste from a can, freeze the remaining paste for up to three months in single serving sizes, or 1 to 2 tablespoons, using an ice cube tray or other small mold.

Per serving: Calories: 323; Total fat: 5g; Saturated fat: 1g; Protein: 18g; Carbohydrates: 55g; Fiber: 18g; Sodium: 597mg

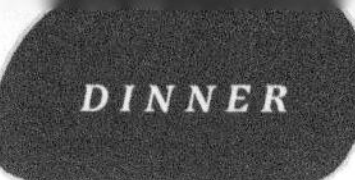

White Bean and Artichoke Stew

30-MINUTE, ONE-POT

SERVES	PREP TIME	COOK TIME
4	5 minutes	25 minutes

Artichokes are one of the highest-ranked vegetables for antioxidant content and are rich in fiber, potassium, vitamin C, and folate. In this quick stew, they add their notable buttery flavor to create an easy and delicious weeknight meal. To save on time even further, use about 4 cups of packaged fresh baby kale leaves in place of the bunch.

- 4 cups vegetable broth
- 1 (15-ounce) can artichoke hearts, drained and chopped
- 1 (15-ounce) can diced tomatoes
- 1 (15-ounce) can white beans, drained and rinsed
- 1 teaspoon dried basil
- 1 teaspoon dried oregano
- 1 teaspoon sea salt
- 1 bunch kale, stemmed and chopped
- ¼ cup shredded Parmesan cheese, for serving

1. In a large pot, combine the broth, artichoke hearts, tomatoes and their juices, beans, basil, oregano, and salt. Bring to a boil over high heat, then reduce the heat to medium-low and simmer for 15 minutes, until the flavors meld.
2. Add the kale and cook for 5 more minutes, until softened. Serve topped with Parmesan cheese.

Ingredient tip: If you have fresh herbs on hand, use those instead. Use 1 tablespoon each of chopped basil and oregano leaves.

Per serving: Calories: 218; Total fat: 2g; Saturated fat: 1g; Protein: 13g; Carbohydrates: 36g; Fiber: 11g; Sodium: 1,669mg

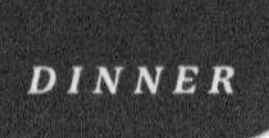

Eggplant, Tofu, and Edamame Stir-Fry

30-MINUTE, ONE-PAN

SERVES	PREP TIME	COOK TIME
4	10 minutes	15 minutes

Eggplant and tofu take on the flavor of whatever you cook them with, and both are nutritional powerhouses, making them wonderful additions to a stir-fry. Eggplant is rich in fiber, and potassium, while tofu is a great source of protein. The edamame, which are immature soybeans, add a nice green touch and an additional bit of fiber and protein.

1 pound Japanese eggplant, cut into 1-inch cubes

1 teaspoon sea salt, divided

8 ounces firm tofu

1 tablespoon toasted sesame oil

½ cup chopped scallions, white and green parts, divided

3 garlic cloves, minced

1 cup frozen shelled edamame, thawed

1 tablespoon sesame seeds, for serving

1. In a colander, sprinkle the eggplant with ½ teaspoon of salt and set over the sink to drain. After about 5 minutes, squeeze the eggplant to extract as much water as possible.
2. While the eggplant drains, slice the tofu into horizontal slabs. Using a clean kitchen towel, press each slab to remove as much water as possible. Cut into 1-inch cubes.
3. In a large skillet, heat the oil over medium-high heat. Sauté the white parts of the scallions and the garlic for 30 seconds, until fragrant. Add the eggplant and sauté for about 5 minutes, stirring regularly, until browned.
4. Add the tofu to the pan and sauté for 5 more minutes, until browned, stirring regularly to prevent burning. Stir in the edamame, add the remaining ½ teaspoon of salt, and cook for 2 more minutes, until the edamame is heated through.
5. Stir the remaining scallion greens into the skillet and serve topped with sesame seeds.

Ingredient tip: Japanese eggplant are thin and small compared to the Italian variety. I like to use them instead of globe eggplant for their higher skin-to-flesh ratio, which works well in a stir-fry—the skin is able to crisp during cooking, adding a nice texture to the dish. If you can't find them, you can use any other variety instead.

FODMAP-Friendly tip: Replace the tofu and edamame with your favorite protein source, use the green part of the scallions only, and use Onion-and-Garlic-Infused Oil (see page 61) instead of fresh garlic.

Per serving: Calories: 169; Total fat: 8g; Saturated fat: 1g; Protein: 11g; Carbohydrates: 14g; Fiber: 6g; Sodium: 606mg

Lentil Curry with Sweet Potatoes and Raita

SERVES	PREP TIME	COOK TIME
4 to 6	10 minutes	30 minutes

Lentils are highly nutritious, but one of the best things about them is how quickly they cook. Unlike other beans and legumes that require soaking, lentils cook easily and are perfect instruments for seasoning with the warm and comforting flavors of curry and coconut milk.

1 tablespoon extra-virgin olive oil

1 yellow onion, chopped

2 garlic cloves, minced

½ inch fresh ginger root, peeled and minced

1 cup brown lentils

1 large sweet potato, chopped

1 teaspoon ground turmeric

1 teaspoon curry power

3½ cups water

1 cup full-fat coconut milk

1 teaspoon sea salt, plus more for seasoning

1 cup coconut milk yogurt

½ cucumber, seeded and grated

½ teaspoon ground cumin

Cooked brown rice, quinoa, millet, or cauliflower rice, for serving

1. In a large pot, heat the oil over medium heat. Add the onion and cook for 3 to 5 minutes, until softened. Add the garlic and ginger and cook for about 1 minute, until fragrant.
2. Add the lentils, sweet potato, turmeric, and curry powder. Stir well to combine and pour the water into the pot to cover the lentils and sweet potatoes. Bring to a boil, reduce the heat, and simmer for 20 minutes, until the lentils and sweet potato are tender. Stir in the coconut milk and salt.
3. Meanwhile in a small bowl, combine the coconut milk yogurt, cucumber, and cumin and mix well. Season with salt.
4. Serve the curry over brown rice with the yogurt-cucumber mixture (raita) on the side.

FODMAP-Friendly tip: Omit the onions and garlic in step 1 and instead use onion-and-garlic infused oil when sautéing the ginger.

Per serving: Calories (without rice): 393; Total fat: 18g; Saturated fat: 12g; Protein: 15g; Carbohydrates: 46g; Fiber: 17g; Sodium: 618mg

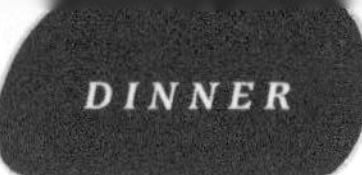

Mediterranean Quinoa Salad

30-MINUTE, LOW-FODMAP

SERVES	PREP TIME	COOK TIME
4	10 minutes	20 minutes

Quinoa is perfect in this salad as it soaks up the dressing without turning mushy and holds up perfectly in the refrigerator for up to five days, making this a great meal to plan ahead. Use lightly sautéed tofu in place of chicken for a plant-based alternative.

- 1 pound boneless, skinless chicken breasts, halved lengthwise
- Juice of 2 lemons, divided
- 3 tablespoons extra-virgin olive oil, divided
- 1 teaspoon dried basil
- 1 teaspoon dried oregano
- Sea salt
- Freshly ground black pepper
- 2 cups water
- 1 cup quinoa
- 1 (15-ounce) can chickpeas or white beans
- 1 cucumber, peeled and finely chopped
- 1 red bell pepper, finely chopped
- 1 bunch parsley, leaves finely chopped

1. In a bowl, combine the chicken, juice of 1 lemon, 1 tablespoon of oil, basil, and oregano and mix. Season with salt and pepper and set aside.
2. In a small pot, combine the water and quinoa and bring to a boil over medium-high heat. Reduce the heat and simmer until the water is nearly absorbed, about 10 minutes. Cover the pot, turn off the heat, and let steam for 5 minutes.
3. Meanwhile, in a large bowl, toss the chickpeas, cucumber, bell pepper, parsley, the remaining juice of 1 lemon, and the remaining 2 tablespoons of oil. Season with salt and pepper. When the quinoa is done, toss it with the chickpea salad.
4. While the quinoa is cooking, heat a large skillet over medium-high heat. Add the chicken and its marinade to the pan and cook for 3 to 5 minutes, until browned. Flip and continue to cook for 3 to 5 minutes more, until cooked through. Let rest for 5 minutes, then slice and serve over the chickpea-quinoa salad.

Per serving: Calories: 512; Total fat: 17g; Saturated fat: 2g; Protein: 36g; Carbohydrates: 59g; Fiber: 10g; Sodium: 314mg

Whitefish in Parchment with Vegetables

30-MINUTE, LOW-FODMAP, ONE-PAN

SERVES	PREP TIME	COOK TIME
4	15 minutes	15 minutes

Parchment-steamed fish packages are quick to throw together, easily customizable, and always tender and juicy. Prepare them the night before and store in the refrigerator to pop in the oven when you get home from work, and dinner will be ready in no time. Here are two variations.

For the tamari-ginger whitefish

1 large bok choy head, sliced into ½-inch strips

1 red bell pepper, sliced

1 pound whitefish fillets (cod, sole, tilapia)

4 scallions, white and green parts, cut into 3-inch segments

3 inches fresh ginger root, peeled and julienned

Sea salt

Freshly ground black pepper

3 tablespoons tamari

Juice of 1 lime

Cooked brown rice, quinoa, or millet, for serving

For the lemon-pepper whitefish

2 medium zucchini, sliced

1 medium carrot, cut into thin strips

1 pound whitefish fillets (cod, sole, tilapia)

4 scallions, white and green parts, cut into 3-inch segments

Sea salt

Freshly ground black pepper

Grated zest and juice of 1 lemon

Cooked brown rice, quinoa, or millet, for serving

To make the tamari-ginger whitefish

1. Preheat the oven to 400°F.
2. Cut 4 (12-inch square) pieces of parchment paper.
3. On one piece of parchment paper, place one-quarter of the bok choy and red peppers and lay a fish fillet on top. Place one-quarter of the scallions and ginger on top and lightly season with salt and pepper. Repeat with remaining paper, fish, and vegetables.
4. In a small bowl, combine the tamari and lime juice and divide evenly over the fish.

5. Fold the parchment over the top of the fish and vegetables and crease along the edges to form packets. Place the finished packets on a large baking sheet.
6. Bake for 10 to 12 minutes for thinner fillets, or up to 16 minutes for thicker fillets. Open carefully to allow the steam to escape, then serve over a bed of brown rice.

To make the lemon-pepper whitefish

1. Preheat the oven to 400°F.
2. Cut 4 (12-inch square) pieces of parchment paper.
3. On one piece of parchment paper, place one-quarter of the zucchini and carrots and lay a fish fillet on top. Place one-quarter of the scallions and lightly season with salt and pepper. Repeat with remaining paper, fish, and vegetables.
4. Sprinkle the lemon zest over the fillets and divide the lemon juice over top of the fish. Finish with more freshly ground black pepper.
5. Fold the parchment over the top of the fish and vegetables and crease along the edges to form packets. Place the finished packets on a large baking sheet.
6. Bake for 10 to 12 minutes for thinner fillets, or up to 16 minutes for thicker fillets. Open carefully to allow the steam to escape, then serve over a bed of brown rice.

Preparation tip: If you don't have parchment paper, use aluminum foil instead.

Tamari-Ginger Whitefish (without rice): Per serving: Calories: 152; Total fat: 1g; Saturated fat: <1g; Protein: 29g; Carbohydrates: 6g; Fiber: 1g; Sodium: 881mg

Lemon-Pepper Whitefish (without rice): Per serving: Calories: 149; Total fat: 1g; Saturated fat: <1g; Protein: 27g; Carbohydrates: 7g; Fiber: 2g; Sodium: 111mg

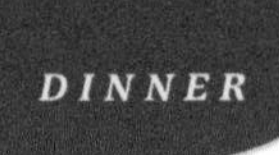

DINNER

Thai Fish Stew

30-MINUTE, ONE-POT

SERVES	PREP TIME	COOK TIME
4	15 minutes	15 minutes

Thai curry has a luxurious flavor and aroma, created by the combination of salty, sweet, and spice in this coconut-based stew. Here, green beans bulk up the stew for a healthy, fiber-filled meal. To make it even heartier, add a cup of zucchini noodles to each bowl, then spoon the stew over the top.

- 1 (13.5-ounce) can full-fat coconut milk, divided
- 2 tablespoons Thai red curry paste
- 3 garlic cloves, minced
- 3 cups vegetable broth or Bone Broth (page 139)
- 12 ounces whitefish fillets
- 2 cups trimmed green beans
- 2 Roma tomatoes, cut into 1-inch pieces
- ½ cup sliced white mushrooms (optional)
- 2 tablespoons fish sauce
- 1 tablespoon coconut sugar (optional)
- Juice of 1 lime
- ½ cup chopped fresh cilantro, for serving

1. In a large pot, heat the cream from the top of the coconut milk over medium heat until melted. Stir in the curry paste and garlic and cook for 1 minute, until fragrant.
2. Pour about 1 cup of broth into the pot and stir with the curry mixture to combine. Add the remaining 2 cups of broth and the remaining coconut milk and stir. Bring to a simmer.
3. Add the fish to the pot, cover, and cook for 5 minutes, until the fish is nearly done.
4. Add the green beans, tomatoes, and mushrooms (if using) and simmer for 5 more minutes, until the vegetables are tender and the fish flakes with a fork.
5. Add the fish sauce, coconut sugar (if using), and lime juice. Taste and season with additional fish sauce or lime juice, if desired. Serve with cilantro.

FODMAP-Friendly tip: Omit the mushrooms or replace with red peppers.

Per serving: Calories: 328; Total fat: 19g; Saturated fat: 15g; Protein: 23g; Carbohydrates: 15g; Fiber: 3g; Sodium: 1,329mg

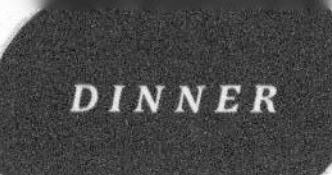

Sheet Pan Salmon with Sweet Potatoes and Brussels Sprouts

30-MINUTE

SERVES	PREP TIME	COOK TIME
4	10 minutes	20 minutes

Salmon is one of the easiest sheet pan meals out there because of its quick cooking time. While you can peel the sweet potato if you prefer, I like to leave the skin on to get the added benefit of the extra fiber. The three-ingredient marinade featuring miso is a great way to use this flavorful, probiotic-filled condiment.

- 2 tablespoons white miso
- 2 tablespoons tamari
- 1 teaspoon toasted sesame oil
- 1 pound salmon fillet
- 2 sweet potatoes, cut into ½-inch cubes
- 1 tablespoon extra-virgin olive oil, divided
- Sea salt
- Freshly ground black pepper
- 1 pound Brussels sprouts, trimmed and halved

1. Preheat the oven to 400°F.
2. In a large dish, combine the miso, tamari, and sesame oil. Place the salmon, skin-side down, in the miso mixture.
3. In a large bowl, toss the sweet potatoes with 1½ teaspoons of the olive oil and season with salt and pepper. Spread the potatoes on the baking sheet around the salmon. In the same bowl, toss the Brussels sprouts with the remaining 1½ teaspoons of olive oil and spread them around the salmon.
4. Bake for 15 to 20 minutes, until the salmon is cooked through and flakes easily with a fork and the sweet potatoes and Brussels sprouts are tender. Serve.

Variation tip: Leftover sweet potatoes and Brussels sprouts make a great breakfast hash the next day. Heat them in a skillet to warm through. Fry one or two eggs and serve over top of the vegetables for a quick, nutritious meal.

FODMAP-Friendly tip: Swap out the Brussels sprouts for broccoli or collard greens.

Per serving: Calories: 317; Total fat: 10g; Saturated fat: 2g; Protein: 29g; Carbohydrates: 29g; Fiber: 6g; Sodium: 865mg

One-Pot Chicken with Jerusalem Artichokes and Potatoes

ONE-POT

SERVES	PREP TIME	COOK TIME
4	10 minutes	30 minutes

Jerusalem artichokes are naturally rich in inulin, which can help improve digestive function. Here they are cooked alongside potatoes for this comfort-food classic of braised chicken. Scented with rosemary, this fragrant chicken will always turn out juicy with just a little help from you in this easy one-pot method.

- 2 tablespoons extra-virgin olive oil, divided
- 4 bone-in chicken thighs
- ¾ teaspoons sea salt
- ½ teaspoon freshly ground black pepper
- 8 ounces small red or purple potatoes, cut into 1-inch pieces
- 8 ounces Jerusalem artichokes, peeled and cut into 1-inch pieces
- 1 cup chicken broth or Bone Broth (page 139)
- 2 rosemary sprigs

1. Preheat the oven to 400°F.
2. In a large cast-iron skillet, heat 1 tablespoon of oil over medium-high heat. Season the chicken with the salt and pepper and place it, skin-side down, in the oil to cook for 3 to 5 minutes, until it is browned and easily releases from the pan. Flip the chicken over and cook for an additional 3 minutes, until browned. Remove the chicken from the pan and set aside.
3. In the same skillet, heat the remaining 1 tablespoon of oil over medium-high heat. Add the potatoes and artichokes and cook for 3 to 5 minutes, until just lightly browned. Add the chicken back into the skillet between the artichokes and potatoes. Pour in the broth and add the rosemary.
4. Transfer the skillet to the oven and bake for 10 to 15 minutes, until the vegetables are tender and the chicken is cooked through and juices run clear. Serve.

FODMAP-Friendly tip: Swap out the Jerusalem artichokes for carrots.

Per serving: Calories: 393; Total fat: 26g; Saturated fat: 6g; Protein: 22g; Carbohydrates: 19g; Fiber: 2g; Sodium: 590mg

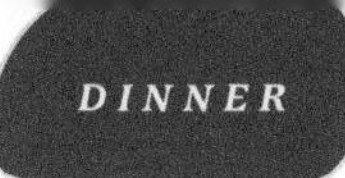

Miso-Tamari Soba Noodles with Chicken

30-MINUTE

SERVES	PREP TIME	COOK TIME
4	10 minutes	20 minutes

Buckwheat soba noodles are hearty and filling and have a great nutty flavor that pairs well with miso-tamari sauce in this easy weeknight noodle dish. Miso is a versatile ingredient that can add a probiotic boost to many foods—just a little goes a long way for a lot of flavor.

1 large boneless, skinless chicken breast, halved lengthwise

8 ounces buckwheat soba noodles

¼ cup sesame seeds

2 teaspoons tamari

2 teaspoons miso paste

1 tablespoon toasted sesame oil

1 cup frozen shelled edamame, thawed

1 carrot, shaved with a vegetable peeler

4 scallions, white and green parts, thinly sliced

1. Place the chicken in a small pot and cover with a couple of inches of water. Bring to a boil over medium-high heat, then reduce the heat to low and cover. Cook for about 8 minutes, until the chicken is cooked through and the juices run clear. Remove the chicken from the poaching liquid, reserving the liquid, and set aside.
2. Bring a large pot of water to a boil over high heat and cook the buckwheat soba according to package directions. Drain and transfer to a large bowl.
3. In a high-speed blender, combine the sesame seeds, tamari, miso, and oil and blend well. Add 2 to 3 tablespoons of the poaching liquid and blend to create a smooth sauce.
4. Using two forks, shred the chicken and toss in a bowl with the noodles, edamame, carrot, and scallions. Pour the sauce over top and toss.

FODMAP-Friendly tip: Don't use the white parts of the scallions, omit the edamame, and double up on the carrots instead.

Per serving: Calories: 407; Total fat: 12g; Saturated fat: 2g; Protein: 27g; Carbohydrates: 48g; Fiber: 4g; Sodium: 27g

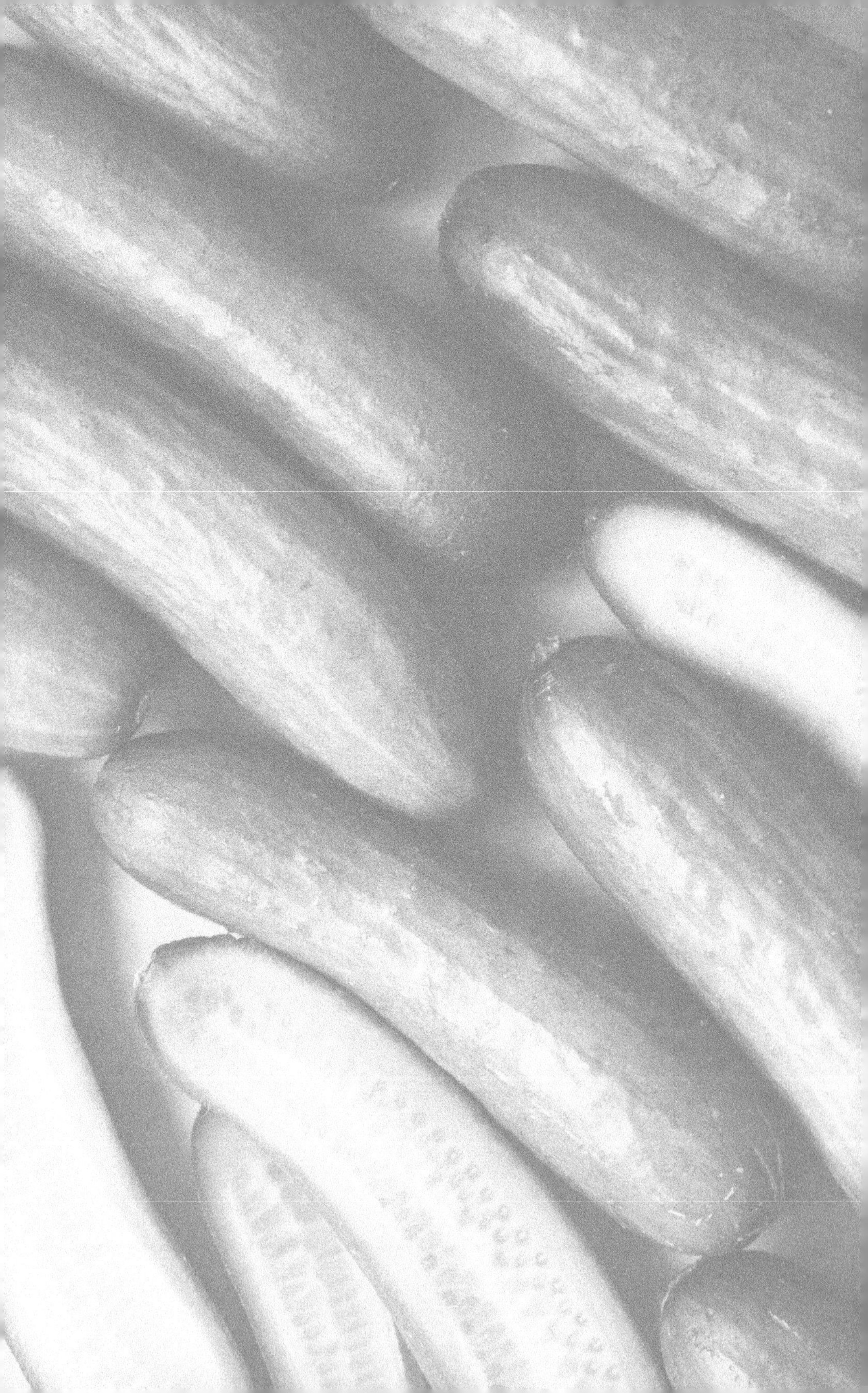

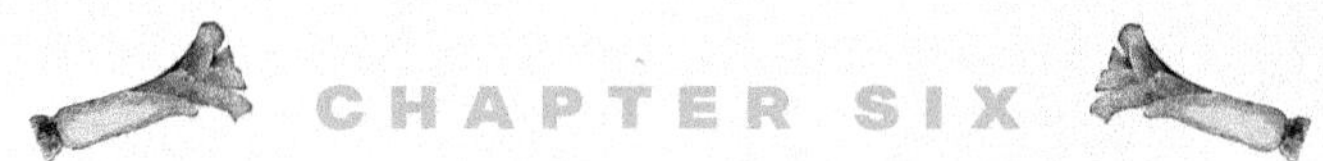

CHAPTER SIX

Recipes for Probiotic-Filled Fermented Foods

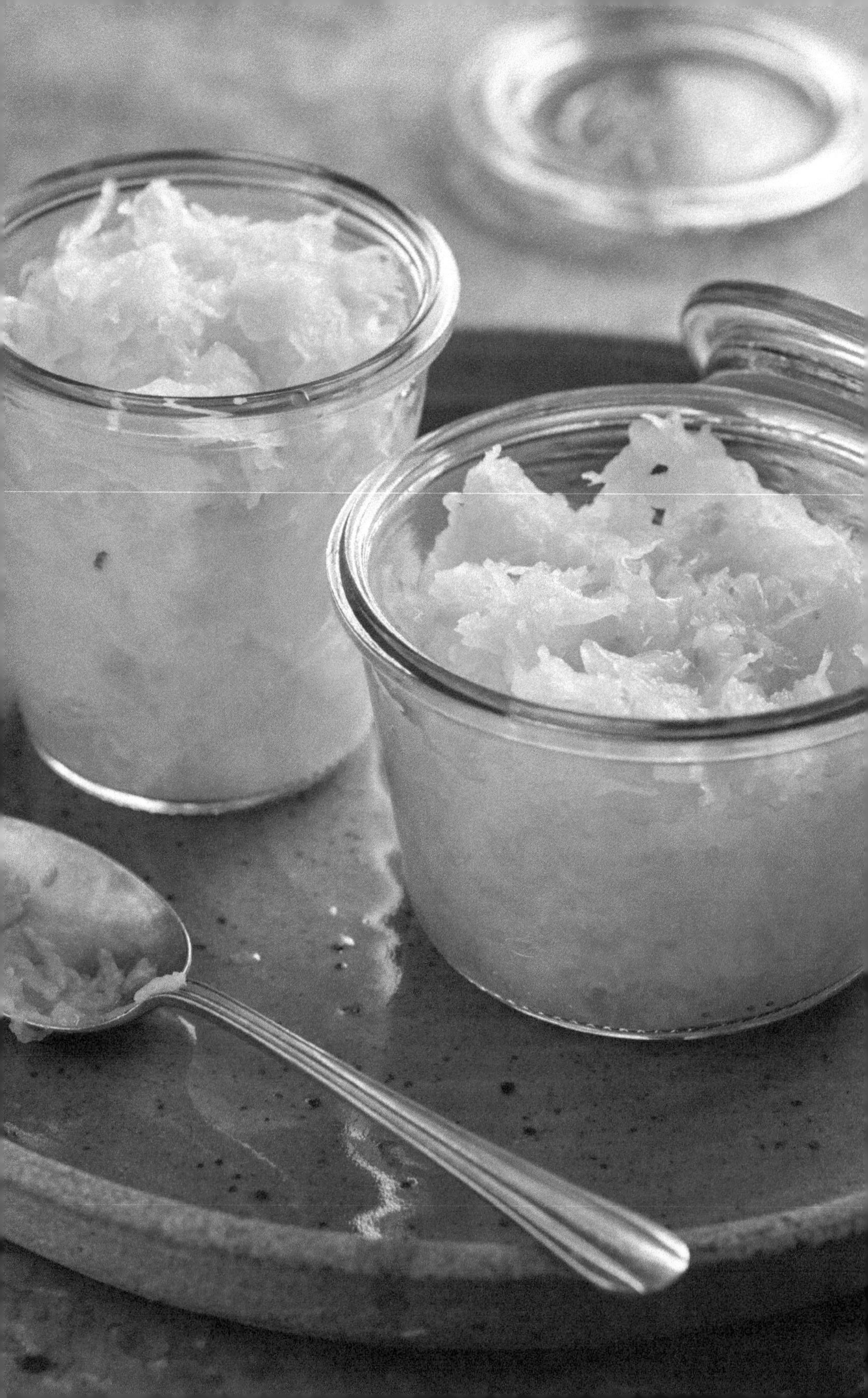

Sauerkraut

MAKES	PREP TIME	FERMENTATION TIME
1 quart	10 minutes	5 to 14 days

Sauerkraut is perfect for your first try at fermentation. Loaded with vitamin C, the anti-inflammatory amino acid glutamine, and anticarcinogenic glucosinolates, cabbage actually increases in nutritional value through fermentation and has the potential benefit of strengthening the immune system. Skip the pricey artisanal ferments and make this simple classic with just a head of cabbage and salt. The keys are using your hands to mix the salt and cabbage to ensure it is evenly coated and holding the cabbage below the brine in an anaerobic environment.

1 (2 to 3 pound) cabbage head, shredded

1½ tablespoons sea salt

1. In a large bowl, combine the salt and cabbage and use your hands to mix well. Let rest at room temperature for 30 minutes, until slightly wilted and some water is released.
2. Tightly pack the cabbage into a quart jar, pressing down with your fist. Pour any accumulated water into the jar.
3. Close the jar loosely with a lid and leave at room temperature overnight. By the following day, the brine should cover the vegetables. If it hasn't, mix 1 cup of water with 1 teaspoon of salt and pour into the jar to cover the cabbage.
4. Use a weight to hold the cabbage down below the brine. Cover the jar loosely with a lid, an airlock, or a tightly woven cloth secured by a rubber band and ferment in a cool location for 5 to 14 days. If using a lid, open the jar daily to allow gases to escape. After 5 days, begin tasting the sauerkraut. When it is soured to your liking, remove the weight, tightly close the jar with a lid, and transfer it to the refrigerator to halt fermentation. Store for up to several months.

Ingredient tip: Be sure to look for sea salt that does not have any other ingredients in it. Many varieties of salt are iodized or have other anticaking agents that can interfere with fermentation, so finding pure salt is important.

Fermented Radishes

MAKES	PREP TIME	FERMENTATION TIME
1 quart	10 minutes	2 to 5 days

Cultured radishes take on a great texture, look lovely in the jar, and are a good source of vitamin C, potassium, folic acid, vitamin B_6, magnesium, copper, and calcium. This simple ferment is ready in just a few days, depending on how soured you want the radishes. Begin tasting these early, as radishes tend to soften quickly. Fermented radishes go great on salads, pair nicely with chicken, and taste amazing straight out of the jar.

- 4 cups water
- 2 tablespoons sea salt
- 1 teaspoon mustard seeds
- 2 bunches radishes, tops and bottoms trimmed, cut into quarters

1. In a bowl, combine the water and salt, stirring until the salt is completely dissolved. Set the brine aside.
2. Place the mustard seeds in a quart jar. Pack the radishes tightly into the jar and pour the brine into the jar, leaving 1 inch of space at the top. Use a weight, if needed, to hold the radishes below the surface of the brine.
3. Cover the jar with a tight lid, an airlock, or a tightly woven cloth secured by a rubber band and set at room temperature to ferment for 2 to 5 days, until the desired flavor is achieved. If using a lid, open the jar daily to allow gases to escape.
4. When finished, close the jar with a tight lid, transfer to the refrigerator, and store for several weeks.

Ingredient tip: If you are using a coarse salt, it may be necessary to heat the water to dissolve it. To do this, heat 1 cup of water, stir in the salt until dissolved, and add the remaining 3 cups of water. Cool to room temperature before using.

Fermented Turnips

MAKES	PREP TIME	FERMENTATION TIME
1 quart	10 minutes	3 to 5 days

Raw turnips can be pungent and strong, but when fermented, turnips, like radishes, lose some of their bite and transform into deliciousness. Turnips are a digestive aid similar to radishes and are particularly high in anticarcinogenic glucosinolates, as well as being a good source of vitamin C. Red pepper flakes add a bit of heat to this blend, but if you cannot tolerate the spice, feel free to omit them.

3 cups water
1½ tablespoons sea salt
2 garlic cloves, peeled
1 teaspoon red pepper flakes
6 medium turnips, sliced

1. In a bowl, combine the water and salt and stir until the salt is dissolved. Set the brine aside.
2. Place the garlic and red pepper flakes in a quart jar. Tightly pack the turnips into the jar and pour the brine over the turnips, leaving about 1 inch of space at the top. Use a weight, if needed, to hold the turnips below the surface of the brine.
3. Close the jar with a tight lid, an airlock, or a tightly woven towel secured by a rubber band. Ferment at room temperature for 3 to 5 days, until it reaches your preferred flavor. If using a lid, open the jar daily to allow gases to escape.
4. When finished, close the jar with a tight lid, transfer to the refrigerator, and store for several weeks.

Preparation tip: Weights are important to hold vegetables below the brine and create an anaerobic environment for lactic acid fermentation. Some weights that can be used include a cleaned rock, a small glass that sits inside the jar, or weights specially designed for this purpose. Whatever you use, it should be cleaned very well and should not be plastic or metal.

Gingered Beets and Carrots

MAKES	PREP TIME	FERMENTATION TIME
1 quart	10 minutes	7 to 10 days

When you are fermenting beets, you want to look for fresh, young beets, preferably with their greens still attached, as this is a sign of freshness. Old fibrous beets will not transform into tender fermented ones, but young ones will be sublime. Ginger helps soothe the stomach, and beets contain the potent anticarcinogen betacyanin, folate, potassium, and iron, making this blend as good for your body as it is delicious.

1 tablespoon minced or grated fresh ginger root

2 medium beets, peeled and shredded

2 carrots, shredded

2 cups water

1 tablespoon sea salt

1. Place the ginger on the bottom of a quart jar, then pack the beets and carrots into the jar.
2. In a bowl, combine the water and salt and stir until the salt is dissolved. Pour this brine over the beets to cover, leaving 1 inch of space at the top. Use a weight to hold the vegetables below the surface.
3. Close the jar using a tight lid, an airlock, or a tightly woven cloth secured by a rubber band. Ferment at room temperature for 7 to 10 days, until the flavor is to your liking. If using a lid, open the jar daily to allow gases to escape.
4. When finished, close the jar with a tight lid, transfer to the refrigerator, and store for several weeks.

Kimchi

MAKES	PREP TIME	FERMENTATION TIME
1 quart	10 minutes	3 to 14 days

A cousin of sauerkraut, kimchi is a spicy pickled condiment hailing from Korea and made using Napa cabbage. In this recipe, daikon and carrots are added for a bit of extra crunch. While this recipe makes about 1 quart of kimchi, ferment it in a larger jar if possible, preferably a half gallon, to prevent the brine from spilling over the top during fermentation.

- 3 tablespoons sea salt, plus 1½ teaspoons
- 4 cups water
- 1 pound daikon, sliced
- 2 carrots, thinly sliced
- ½ Napa cabbage head, cut into 1-inch cubes
- 2 scallions, white and green parts, cut into 1-inch segments
- 3 garlic cloves, crushed
- 1 inch fresh ginger root, peeled and cut into matchsticks
- 2 tablespoons Korean ground red pepper

1. In a large bowl, combine 3 tablespoons of salt with the water and stir to dissolve. Add the daikon, carrot, and cabbage to the bowl and cover with a plate to hold the vegetables below the brine. Let the mixture rest overnight, or for about 8 hours, at room temperature.
2. The next day, strain the brine from the vegetables, reserving the brine, and return the vegetables to the bowl.
3. Add the scallions, garlic, ginger, red pepper, and the remaining 1½ teaspoons salt to the vegetables. Toss to mix well. Firmly pack the vegetables into a large jar.
4. Pour the reserved brine over the vegetables, leaving about 1 inch of space at the top. Use a weight to hold the vegetables below the brine and cover loosely with a lid, an airlock, or a tightly woven cloth secured with a rubber band.
5. Ferment at room temperature for 3 days to 2 weeks, tasting occasionally, until the desired sourness is achieved. If using a lid, open the jar daily to allow gases to escape.
6. When finished, close the jar with a tight lid, transfer to the refrigerator, and store for up to 1 month.

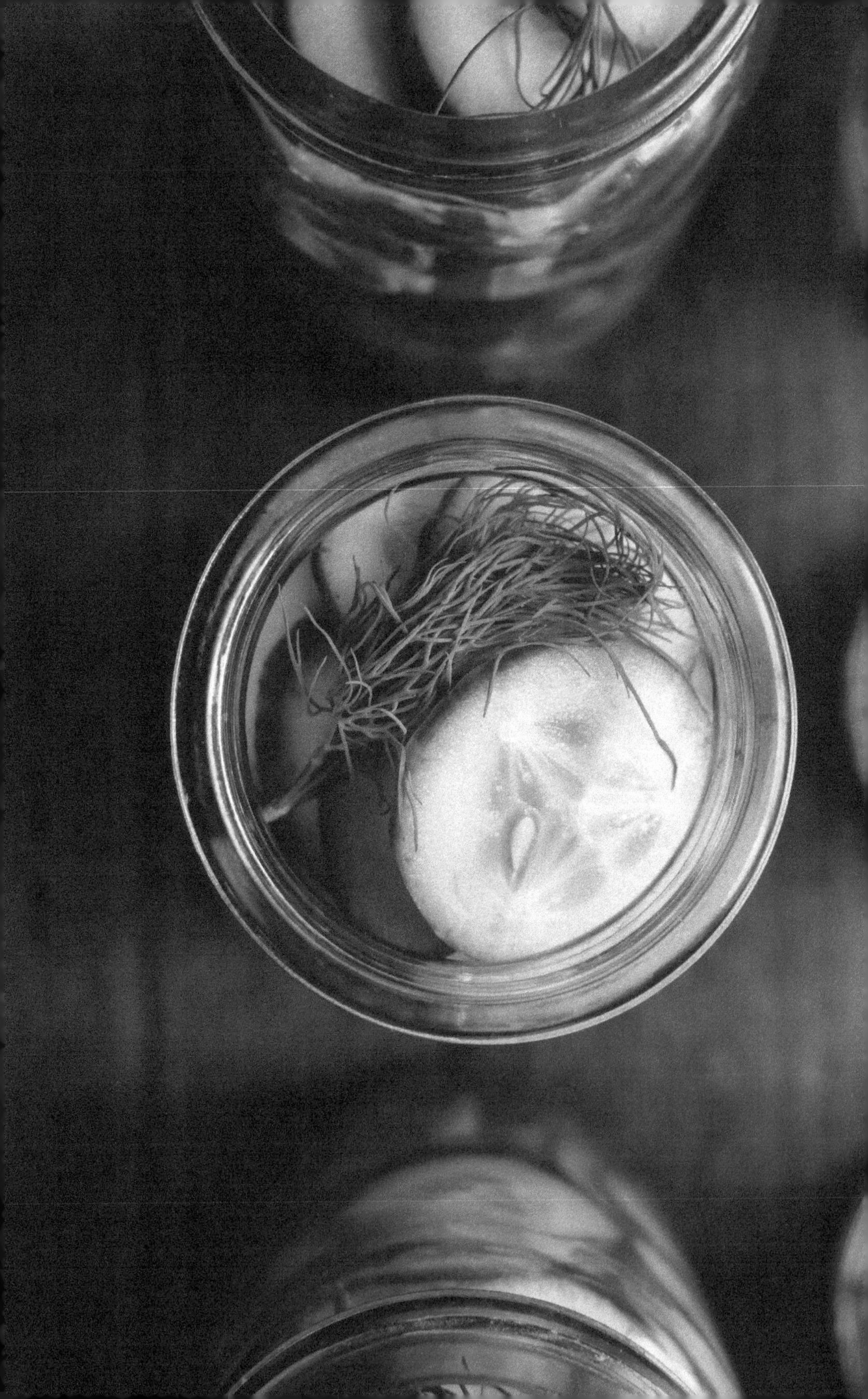

Half-Sour Pickles

MAKES	PREP TIME	FERMENTATION TIME
1 quart	10 minutes	3 to 5 days

Cucumbers are rich in antioxidant and anti-inflammatory phytonutrients, and they are a classic favorite for fermentation. This simple recipe uses everyday spices and salt to create some truly delicious half-sour pickles in just a few days.

- 1 pound pickling cucumbers
- 2 garlic cloves, smashed
- 2 dill heads (optional)
- 6 black peppercorns
- 1 dried red chile
- 4 cups water
- 2 tablespoons sea salt

1. Remove the blossom end of the cucumbers. If desired, quarter or halve the cucumbers lengthwise.
2. Place the garlic, dill heads (if using), peppercorns, and chile into a quart jar. Pack the cucumbers into the jar as tightly as possible.
3. In a bowl, combine the water and salt and stir to dissolve. Pour this brine over the cucumbers, leaving 1 inch of space at the top. Use a weight, if needed, to hold the cucumbers below the brine.
4. Loosely affix a lid, an airlock, or a tightly woven cloth secured with a rubber band and let the cucumbers ferment at room temperature for 3 to 5 days, until the desired sourness is achieved. If using a lid, open the jar daily to allow gases to escape.
5. When finished, close the jar with a tight lid, transfer to the refrigerator, and store for up to 1 month.

Variation tip: Dill heads will give these pickles the classic dill flavor but can be hard to find when not in season. Look for bunches of dill in the summer months, or replace it with 1 tablespoon dill seed or dill weed. Pickling cucumbers are small, less mature cucumbers with small seeds and a firm texture that will hold up during fermentation. Also, they are unwaxed, a necessary component for fermentation. If you are unable to get pickling cucumbers, English cucumbers can be used because they are typically not waxed either but instead are wrapped in plastic—just make sure to cut them into spears before fermentation.

Fermented Salsa

MAKES	PREP TIME	FERMENTATION TIME
1 quart	10 minutes	2 to 4 days

Salsa is a very easy condiment to make, and it tastes even better with the tang of fermentation. Look for a firm variety of tomatoes, like San Marzano or Roma, to keep the water content down, or once cut, let the tomatoes drain over a colander for a few minutes before mixing with the remaining ingredients. Tomatoes are rich in vitamin C and antioxidants, while bell peppers are an excellent source of vitamin C, beta-carotene, vitamin K, and folate.

- 2 pounds tomatoes, chopped
- 1 red bell pepper, chopped
- 1 medium red onion, chopped
- 1 jalapeño pepper, seeded and minced
- 1 garlic clove, minced
- ¼ cup chopped fresh cilantro
- ¼ cup coconut water kefir
- Juice of 1 lime
- 1 teaspoon sea salt

1. In a bowl, combine the tomatoes, bell pepper, onion, jalapeño, garlic, and cilantro. Stir in the kefir, lime juice, and salt.
2. Transfer the mixture to a jar. Use a weight, if needed, to press the vegetables down below the brine. Cover with a tight lid, an airlock, or a tightly woven cloth secured with a rubber band and ferment at room temperature for 2 to 4 days. If using a lid, open the jar daily to allow gases to escape.
3. When finished, close the jar with a tight lid, transfer to the refrigerator, and store for up to 1 month.

Variation tip: If you don't have coconut water kefir on hand, leave it out and increase the salt to 2 teaspoons.

Fermented Ketchup

MAKES	PREP TIME	FERMENTATION TIME
1 pint	10 minutes	2 to 3 days

Using lycopene-rich canned tomato paste, this simple recipe comes together in minutes and is a great alternative to store-bought varieties laden with high-fructose corn syrup and sugar. Fermentation adds loads of healthy bacteria to this condiment, which will be thick and spreadable with a bit of added tang. Sweetened lightly by honey, this blend is a probiotic-rich alternative that goes great with just about anything.

- 2 (6-ounce) cans tomato paste
- 2 tablespoons vinegar
- 2 tablespoons honey
- 2 tablespoons water kefir or brine from fermented vegetables
- ½ teaspoon sea salt
- ¼ teaspoon freshly ground black pepper
- ¼ teaspoon onion powder
- Pinch ground cinnamon
- Pinch ground cloves

1. In a small bowl, combine the tomato paste, vinegar, honey, kefir, salt, pepper, onion powder, cinnamon, and cloves. Taste and adjust seasonings as desired and add water, a little at a time, until the desired consistency is achieved.
2. Cover with a tight lid, an airlock, or a tightly woven cloth secured with a rubber band and leave at room temperature for 2 to 3 days. If using a lid, open the jar daily to allow gases to escape.
3. When finished, close the jar with a tight lid, transfer to the refrigerator, and store for up to 2 months.

Preparation tip: Room temperature is a subjective term, but most ferments typically work best somewhere between 68°F and 72°F. If it is warmer in your house, fermentation will happen more quickly, while if it is cooler, it will take longer. Be sure to check your ferments daily to assess how quickly or slowly they are fermenting and adjust as needed.

Fermented Blackberry Chia Jam

MAKES	PREP TIME
about 1 pint	10 minutes
COOK TIME	**FERMENTATION TIME**
5 minutes	2 days

Chia seeds turn jam-making from a hot, sticky mess to a breeze. They are sticky when soaked, so they work as a thickening agent in place of the more widely used pectin. Chia seeds are also a good source of protein, fiber, antioxidants, and omega-3 fatty acids, making them a perfect addition to your jam.

4 cups blackberries

½ teaspoon sea salt

¼ cup honey

2 tablespoons brine from fermented vegetables

¼ cup chia seeds

1. In a small pot, combine the blackberries and salt. Cook for 5 minutes over medium heat, using the back of a spoon to smash the berries as they soften. Remove the berries from the heat and stir in the honey. Cool to room temperature.
2. Stir in the brine and chia seeds and mix well. Transfer the jam to a clean quart jar and seal tightly with a lid, an airlock, or a tightly woven cloth secured with a rubber band.
3. Ferment at room temperature for 2 days. If using a lid, open the jar daily to allow gases to escape. When finished, close the jar with a tight lid, transfer to the refrigerator, and store for up to 2 months.

Variation tip: Use any combination of berries in this recipe. Raspberries and blueberries both work well in jam. Other ferments such as kombucha or water kefir can be used instead of vegetable brine.

Fauxbucha

MAKES
2 cups

PREP TIME
5 minutes

Kombucha is fabulous. But what if you're not willing to fork over those hard-earned $5 for a 16-ounce bottle? My answer to this vexing issue is fauxbucha! This super-easy-to-make, refreshing concoction tastes like kombucha, offers probiotic pearls from the apple cider vinegar, brings a zingy boost to your immune system from the ginger, and costs a fraction of the price. Look for apple cider vinegar that includes "the mother," which is friendly bacteria and strands of protein that give the vinegar a somewhat cloudy appearance.

- 2 cups water
- 2 inches fresh ginger root, peeled and diced
- ¼ cup apple cider vinegar (with "the mother" in it)
- 1 teaspoon honey or a little stevia
- 1 mint sprig or ginger sliver, for garnish (optional)

1. Put the water, ginger, vinegar, and honey in a blender and blend at high speed for about 30 seconds.
2. Divide the mixture between 2 cups and garnish with a sprig of mint or a sliver of ginger (if using).

Variation tip: You can revise ingredients according to taste.

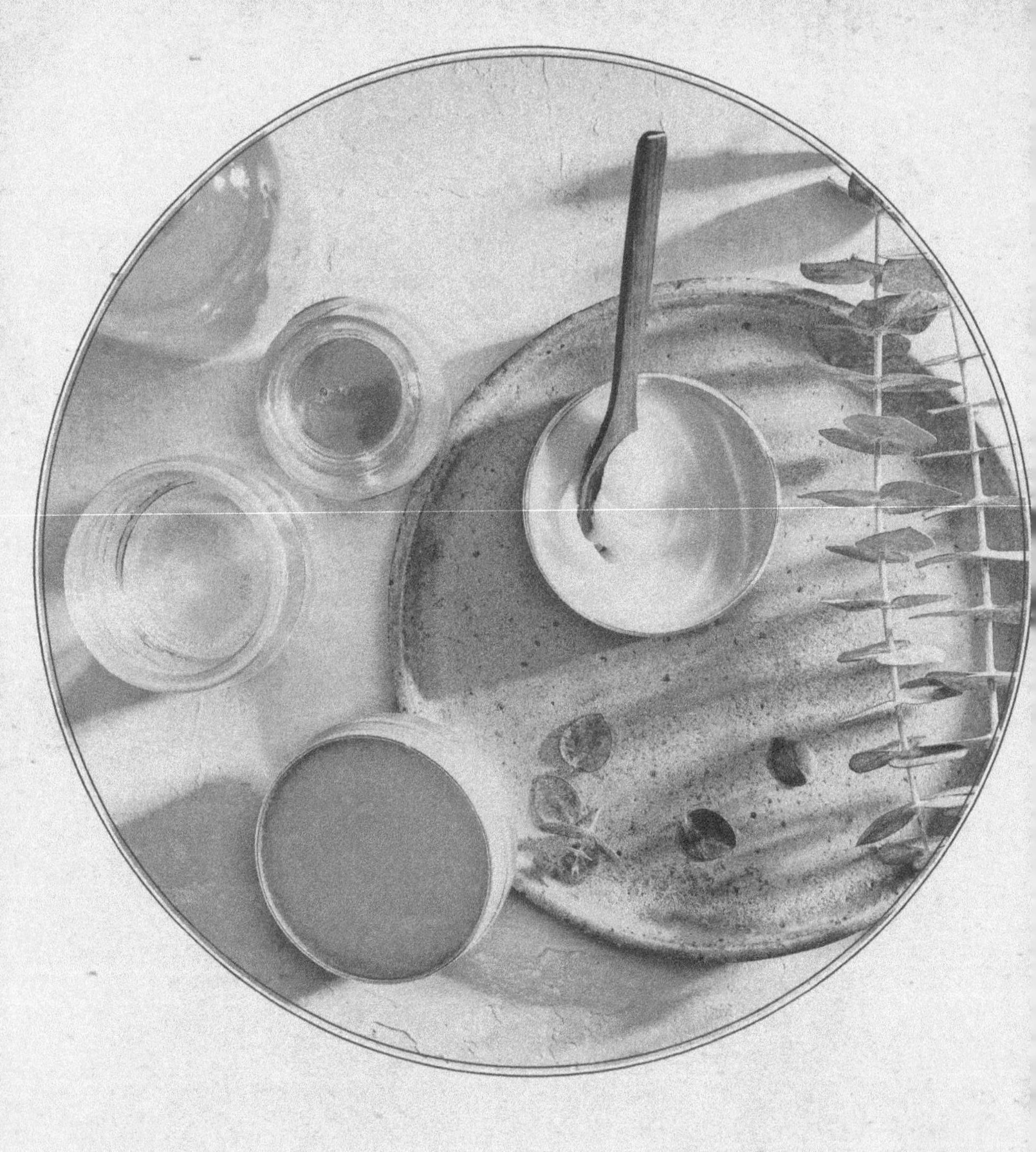

PART THREE

Protect Your Microbiome

WELCOME TO THE Microbiome Task Force. You have committed to preserving and protecting your personal bacterial population. Here are some realistic and practical ways to make that happen. Grab your badge, get out your notebook, contact a friend who likes to keep you accountable, and let's do this.

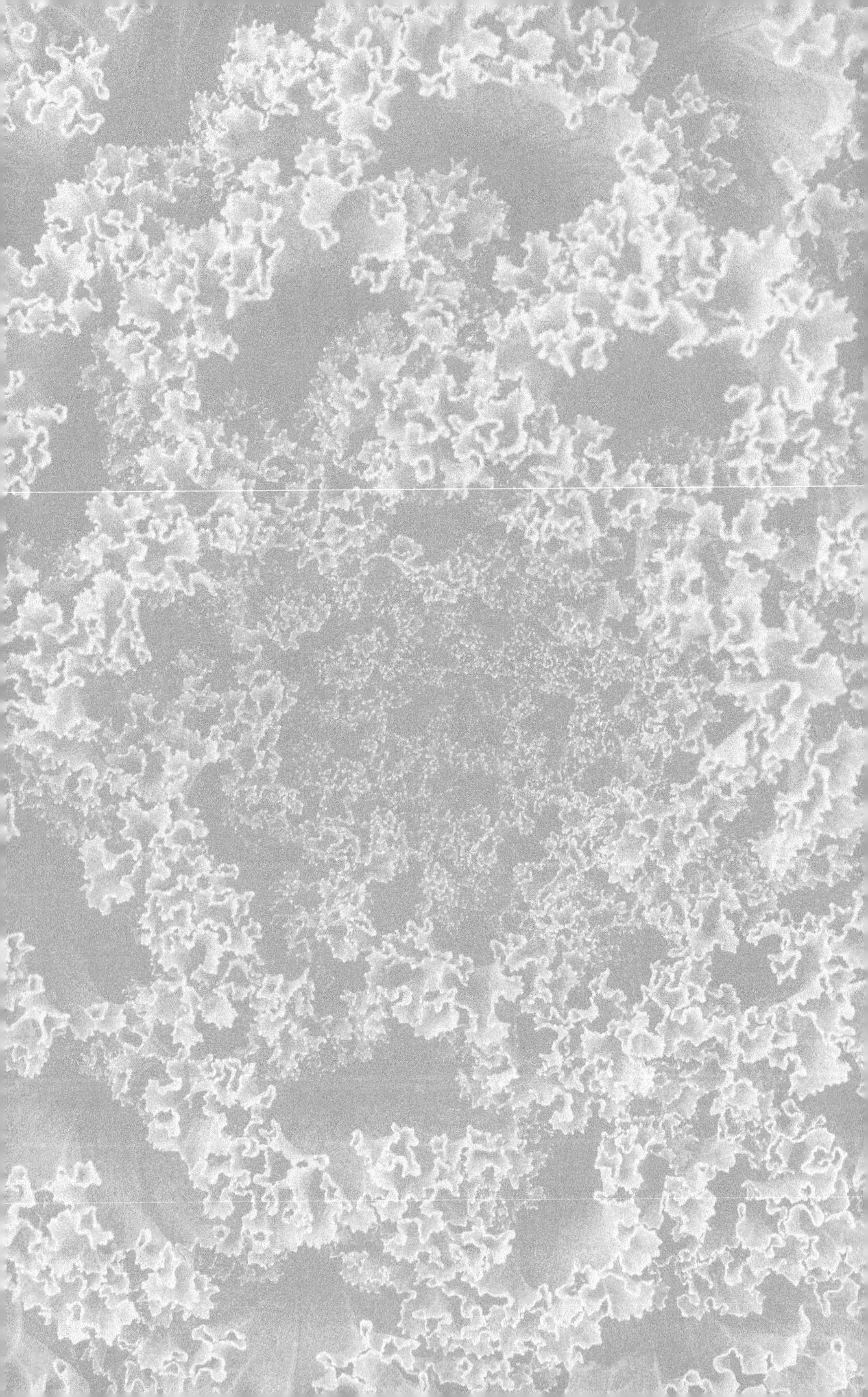

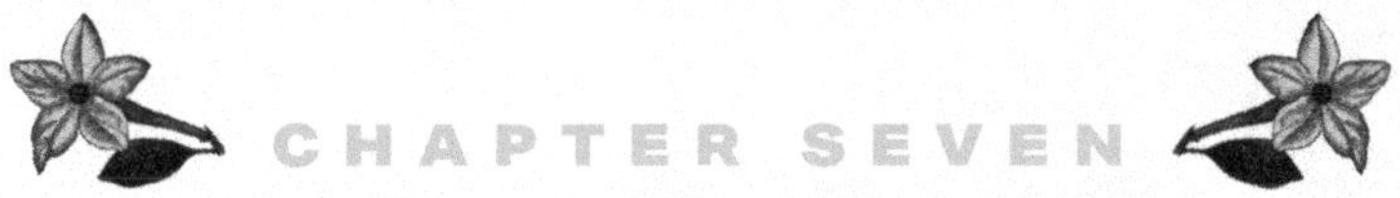

CHAPTER SEVEN

Support Microbial Diversity

Your first mission is to do all you can to support the diversity of your microbiome. This involves breathing some fresh new life into your meals by focusing on gut-healthy ingredients, as well as diversifying your personal activities. Did you ever think that a nap, camping trip, or puppy might be good for the gut? Read on.

Increase Exposure to Diverse Bacteria

Exposing yourself to a variety of microbes is key to gut health. With most things, diversity is what makes us stronger and more resilient.

The idea behind promoting a diverse microbiome is that our bacteria all play different roles and may protect against different pathogens. As such, the more variety of organisms that we have, the more likely it is that our gut will be effective in supporting overall health.

It might make sense then that attaining a diversity of microbes means eating a variety of foods. Eating spinach for breakfast, lunch, and dinner might seem like a good idea, but it will likely mean missing out on a host of other nutrients, as well as the spectrum of those polyphenols that our bugs adore. Different crops are also exposed to different species of bacteria found naturally in the soil. Unless we are rinsing our fruits and vegetables in chlorine or boiling or frying them for extended periods of time, we actually ingest these microscopic bugs every time we munch on an arugula salad or bite into an apple.

Speaking of which, the soil in which your food is grown also makes a difference for gut vitality. Healthy soil should be packed with a variety of microorganisms that protect and defend crops and increase their nutrient value. When we eat foods grown in such soil, we gain all the benefits of that added nourishment. Purchasing organically grown food improves your chances of more nutrient-rich soil having been part of your broccoli's life history. Though it may not be consistent across the board, organic farming practices tend to focus on techniques that enrich and protect the soil. While not everyone has access, if you have the opportunity to buy organic produce, you're doing yourself, the farmers, and the earth a big favor.

In addition to the previously mentioned food-related ideas, the following are some non-food-related ways to diversify your bacterial portfolio:

- You can get that direct exposure to natural bacteria in the soil by spending more time in (you guessed it) nature! Don't be afraid to get a little dirty by getting out into the woods when possible or going for a hike or a camping trip. You may also be able to actually get your hands in the dirt by spending time at a local community garden or by taking your dog (or even your neighbor's dog) for a long walk in the park. Speaking of which . . .

- Spend more time with animals. Whether you are hanging out with a dog, cat, horse, cow, or sheep, some early research indicates that exposure to animal bacteria may have a positive impact on how our bacteria function. That said, following a standard hygiene protocol, including washing your hands afterward, is always a good idea.
- Physical activity is also positively correlated with a more diverse and resilient microbiome, so if there is some way that you love moving your body, whether it's running, biking, playing a group sport, or grooving in your living room, embrace it and find more ways to make that happen. Additional benefits can often include an improved mood, more energy, and a stronger ticker!

And of course, there's the task of maintaining that microbial diversity by engaging in the habits that have been discussed throughout this book: Consume more fiber, fermented foods, and polyphenol-rich foods such as fruits, vegetables, tea, and wine, and eat less sugar, dairy, meat, and processed items. Sound familiar?

Rest and Relax More

Adequate sleep is one of the keys to healthy innards and overall wellness. In fact, recent studies indicate that deeper and longer periods of sleep are associated with a more diverse gut bacteria population. Poor sleep patterns can result in higher levels of inflammation and have the indirect effect of leading us to less optimal food choices. I imagine we've all had days when excessive sleepiness drove us to the candy jar at work. Our slumbering hours are also the time that our bodies heal and regenerate, so skimping on sleep may mean less time for the body to recover and do its important work of keeping us well and repaired from daily stressors. While sleep needs vary from person to person, it's generally recommended that getting a solid seven to nine hours each night can give your body and brain the support it needs. And guess what else? A healthy microbiome has been shown to have positive impacts on sleep. Symbiosis exemplified.

Additionally, your stress can stress out your microbial residents. Have you ever gotten that sinking stomach or wing-flapping butterfly feeling when you feel panicked or under pressure? As with many physiological experiences, there is a mind-body connection going on here. When you experience stress, your body releases hormones in the gut that enable pathogenic, or bad, bacteria to reproduce and promote disrepair and disease. Much research points to a strong connection between high stress and IBS symptoms.

A recent study looked at the effects of various stress management techniques on the microbiota. High stress triggers the "fight or flight response," which prompts the release of a variety of hormones that are meant to be helpful responders. However, these hormones can alter the microbiome when produced in excess. In turn, this disruption can affect the ability of the microbiota to both protect the necessary gut barrier and mediate the feel-good brain chemicals, also known as neurotransmitters.

In particular, meditation has been found to have beneficial effects. While this practice may not be in everyone's comfort zone, it can be worthwhile to engage in some downtime, whether you are in a lotus pose with eyes closed and hands in your lap or simply off your phone for a solid 30 minutes in a relaxing position. Stress management can look different to everyone, so find what works for you and do it more often to assess how it makes a difference.

Just like sleep, stress also has a symbiotic relationship with gut health. Stress may be improved by the presence of a healthy bacterial population, so keeping those bugs happy may be the key to a better stress response. Once again, if you're good to them, they'll be good to you!

It's a good excuse to take a hot bath, lie on the couch to decompress, get that extra hour of sleep tonight, and maybe chant, "Microbi-OMMM."

Minimize Microbial Disruption

Your bacterial community is meant to be a place of peace and harmony, so anything you can do to minimize disruption will be as important as taking all the steps to feed your good bacteria. This means doing what you can to support digestive function, as well as weeding out harmful agents that could be allowing the bad bacteria to take over. As mentioned in chapter 3, there are numerous ways in which your microbes can experience disruption such that their diversity has been reduced, bad bacteria are running amok, and the mucosal barrier lining the intestine has been compromised. All of this can mean impaired immune function.

The following are some ways to counteract common disruptors:

1. **Eschew emulsifiers.** Check the labels of your cartons of alternative milks, ice cream, and other packaged foods to determine how much of these ingredients you consume (see page 33). If you love almond milk, try mixing a teaspoon of almond butter with 8 ounces of water in a blender, and voila: homemade almond milk.
2. **Avoid artificial sweeteners.** This is a good idea generally, but particularly if you want to reduce the chance of microbial imbalance. In place of Splenda or Equal, try maple syrup, honey, and, yes, even a drizzle of molasses for more natural sweetness that also offers a touch of nutritional value. If calories are a concern, it might interest you to know that a teaspoon of these sweeteners has only 15 calories.
3. **Pass on pesticides.** Chemicals found in pesticides have been shown to significantly alter the gut microbiome. If you can't buy organic or pesticide-free produce, you can thoroughly wash it to reduce the residues as much as possible. Dedicated produce wash exists, so seek it out at natural grocery stores.
4. **Sidestep antibacterial soaps and hand gels.** Again, it's always a good idea to practice standard hygiene protocol and wash your hands to avoid passing germs onto others. However, while chemicals in some antibacterial products definitely get rid of the bad germs, they also tend to kill off the helpful ones. Try to avoid products that have a long list of foreign ingredients. Particularly when it comes to sanitizer, a simple alcohol-based version will work just fine.

USING ANTIBIOTICS AND MEDICATION MINDFULLY

Antibiotics saved my dad when he was dealing with a life-threatening infection, so this lady is quite thankful for access to medicines that can save lives and bring her dad back from the hospital.

There are likely many folks who struggle with sinus infections and UTIs who have also praised the antibiotic gods for relieving them of their misery. That being said, antibiotics are often overprescribed (sometimes without even having a definitive diagnosis) and should not be taken frequently if it can be avoided. Just like they sound, antibiotics are anti-BIO (or anti-"life"), meaning that they not only rid your body of the nasty bacteria that cause infections and disease, but they also kill off the beneficial bacteria that you now know are very necessary for optimal human function.

Antibiotics are also often prescribed as a precaution instead of as an intervention and can wind up wreaking havoc over the long run. If you have a serious infection that necessitates an antibiotic, I highly advise you to speak with a physician about a prescription. But fortifying your immune system by strengthening your gut health and not overtaxing your body with stress and poor sleep will increase your body's natural ability to fight off any infections that come your way. Additionally, adding antibacterial herbs, such as thyme, oregano, and rosemary, and immune-supportive foods, such as mushrooms, onions, garlic, ginger, and hot peppers, can help with the fight to prevent infections.

Another common medication that can have detrimental long-term effects on our gut health is acid blockers (also known as "proton pump inhibiters") such as Prilosec and Tagemet. Again, for certain individuals, this medication can be extremely helpful, but in many cases, the medication is addressing symptoms that are occurring because of dietary and lifestyle habits that can be shifted to bring relief. I can't tell you the number of times I've seen a Zantac commercial come right after an Arby's commercial featuring a big beef and gravy sandwich. Coincidence?

If you truly have gastroesophageal reflux disease (GERD), it can be helpful to keep a diet journal to better understand which foods can trigger the sensation of acid reflux. Some common culprits include caffeine, alcohol, chocolate, onions, peppermint, fried and high-fat foods, and general overeating, especially later at night when our digestive fire is slowly dimming. Grazing all day without a break for the stomach can also be a contributing factor. Give yourself a few hours between meals and see how you feel. Also, see the recipe for Ginger Tea Tonic (see page 133) for a way to possibly help reduce symptoms.

Frequent use of laxatives and NSAIDs is also known to be a culprit in microbial disruption. If you are having trouble moving things along internally, take a look at some of our common-remedy recipes in chapter 9. You may find that laxatives are no longer necessary when you consume more fiber and fluids, along with some of the concoctions I've drummed up for you. NSAIDs can also be life savers for those who struggle with chronic pain. Over time, however, they can erode the lining of our stomachs and intestines and increase the likelihood of ulcers. Instead of NSAIDs, heat and meditation have also been shown to have beneficial effects for those who deal with pain regularly. Grab that heating pad or hot-water bottle from the closet and see if you get a little relief.

Finally, antidepressants are shown to have a potentially negative impact on the microbiome. This is not a suggestion to stop taking a medication that may be keeping you balanced—it's more of a reminder that, if you are taking something for mood, it's all the more important that you make it a point to also support your microbial village.

The Difference Between Dirt and Toxicants

A little dirt in your life is a good thing. Research indicates that people who grew up on a farm, played in the dirt, or had animals tend to have a more resilient community of microbes and, as a result, have fewer incidences of ailments such as asthma and allergies. Early exposure to a variety of microorganisms is quite normal and can actually be fortifying to our immune system. It may even be part of the way that our immune system gets educated about the difference between friend and foe. As adults, it is also necessary to have exposure to bacteria in the natural world because it continues to inform and strengthen our immune systems. These days, there is a huge emphasis on hygiene and taking extreme sanitary measures to avoid any kind of exposure to germs. While handwashing is essential for preventing the spread of bad bacteria from one person to another, living in a bubble of antibacterial agents, medical face masks, and rubber gloves could have implications on our microbial health.

Exposure to bacteria in small amounts allows our immune system to identify and build resilience against unfavorable bacteria. There's no need to go around licking doorknobs or sharing utensils with every Tom, Dick, and Harriet you have dinner with, but there may not be a need to fear all foreign bodies. It is, of course, necessary to fear some! There are definitely bad bugs out there, and we do need to be mindful. This is especially true for those who may be more vulnerable to infections—like young children, older adults, and people with a compromised or suppressed immune system.

In particular, immune-compromised individuals may need to pay more attention to cleanliness than the average person. And individuals who have respiratory issues, allergies, or asthma may be particularly sensitive to microbes in the home and other areas where they spend time. Homes can be tested for mold and other harmful bacteria. If you notice an unusual smell or find yourself coughing more when you are in your living space than elsewhere, it might be a good time to hire a specialist to come and assess the scene.

It's also essential that we minimize our exposure to truly unnatural chemical agents found in many common household cleaning products and self-care items, which can have a negative health impact on lung function and may contribute to hormonal disruption. Seek out natural products and avoid high exposure to ingredients that you can't pronounce and that seem like they belong in a chemistry book.

In summary, a little natural dirt in our lives is good. Unwanted microbes and molds, unnatural chemicals, and environmental toxicants are not.

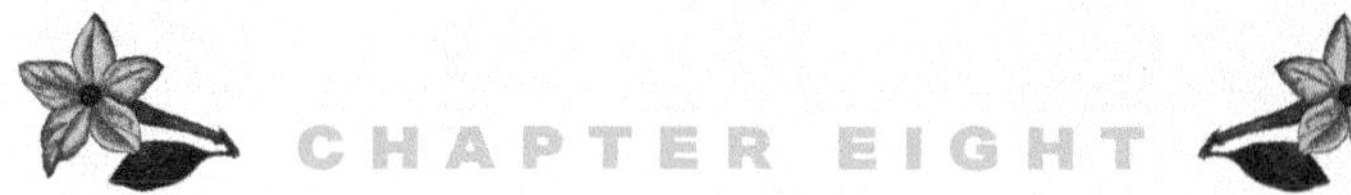

CHAPTER EIGHT

Natural Alternatives to Commercial Cleansers

When was the last time you examined the ingredients in your bathroom cleanser? Chances are, if they are typical commercial products, they contain ingredients that may have negative impacts on our health via the lungs, skin, or mucosal membranes that line our mouth, nostrils, and intestinal tract. While sanitizer use can be critical in certain cases to prevent the spread of germs, many antibacterial cleaning and personal care products can take a toll on your body's friendly microbes. They can also take a toll on your wallet. The following are recipes for gentler and more natural alternatives that can help preserve your financial and bacterial banks!

Mold and Mildew Remover

MAKES
2¼ cups

PREP TIME
5 minutes

Store-bought cleaners may be tough on your skin and lungs, but this simple DIY mixture cuts through both mold and mildew with ease using a few simple household ingredients. Lemon essential oil functions as a disinfectant and antifungal agent, while tea tree essential oil, extracted from a tree native to Australia, has been used for centuries to kill unwanted bacteria, viruses, and fungi. Together, along with vinegar, these powerful oils can be an effective treatment against mold and mildew buildup in the shower and beyond.

1 cup white vinegar

1 cup distilled water

¼ cup isopropyl alcohol

1 teaspoon tea tree essential oil

1 teaspoon lemon essential oil

1. In a spray bottle with a funnel set over top, combine the vinegar, water, and alcohol. Add the essential oils, close the lid, and shake vigorously to mix well.
2. Spray on surfaces and let sit for up to 1 hour before wiping away surface mold and mildew with a brush or cloth.
3. Store in a cool, dark place indefinitely and shake well before each use to disperse the oils.

Tip: Distilled water is made by boiling water into vapor and then collecting the vapor and condensing it back into a liquid, leaving behind any impurities in the water in the original boiling container. This is one method of purification. Distilled water is commonly used in shelf-stable, water-based blends where bacteria growth could be an issue otherwise.

All-Purpose Cleaner

MAKES	PREP TIME
2 cups	5 minutes

Having a functional spray on hand to quickly clean up messes and spills is a must. Use this vinegar-based spray to naturally and safely clean counters and other surfaces as messes happen. The vinegar's acidity cuts through grease and grime to make your surfaces sparkle, and lemon provides disinfectant and antifungal support to make this a great multipurpose cleaner to use throughout the house.

1 cup white vinegar

1 cup distilled water

1 teaspoon lemon essential oil

1. In a spray bottle with a funnel set over top, combine the vinegar, water, and essential oil. Close the lid tightly and shake vigorously to disperse the oils in the liquid.
2. To use, spray on surfaces and let sit for a few minutes, depending on the mess, and wipe up. Repeat if needed.
3. Store in a cool, dark place indefinitely and shake well before each use to disperse the oil.

Tip: Do not use essential oils to clean wood surfaces, as they can strip away the finish on some surfaces.

Scrubbing Cleaner for Shower/Bath

MAKES
½ cup

PREP TIME
5 minutes

Baking soda is one of the most versatile items in your kitchen. Not only is it a wonder for baking, but it is also one of the most effective and cost-effective cleaners you have sitting in your cupboard. Make a batch of this simple scrub in just minutes, and use it to clean your bathroom tile, shower, and tub. Select tea tree, lavender, or lemon essential oils, depending on your preference, or make a mixture using all three.

- ½ cup baking soda
- 10 drops tea tree, lavender, or lemon essential oil
- distilled water, as needed

1. Place the baking soda into a small bowl. Add water, a tablespoon at a time, until a thick paste forms. Add the essential oil and mix well to combine.
2. Spread the paste on bathroom surfaces that need scrubbing, and let it sit for a few minutes before scrubbing with an abrasive pad and rinsing with clean water.

Tip: This mixture does not store well, so it is best made directly before using. It makes enough to clean one standard-size bathtub.

Hand-Cleansing Spray

MAKES
¼ cup

PREP TIME
5 minutes

While washing your hands with soap and water is always the best option, sometimes that is just not possible when you are out and about. Many commercial hand sanitizers, while effective in eliminating germs, are very strongly scented and loaded with chemicals that can negatively affect your healthy microbes. Using antiviral, antifungal, and antibacterial essential oils, along with more natural ingredients, you can quickly create your own hand cleanser that smells great and keeps your hands clean.

5 drops tea tree essential oil

5 drops lavender essential oil

5 drops lemon essential oil

2 tablespoons witch hazel

2 tablespoons distilled water

1. Place a funnel over a 2-ounce, dark-colored spray bottle and pour in the essential oils.
2. Add the witch hazel and fill the bottle with the distilled water. Place the spray nozzle on the bottle tightly and shake well.
3. To use, spray on hands liberally and rub hands together briskly until dry.

Tip: Lemon essential oil can cause photosensitivity, meaning it can increase the effects of the sun on your skin after using. Avoid direct exposure to the sun after using this spray.

Window Cleaner

MAKES
3 cups

PREP TIME
5 minutes

Get streak-free, clean windows with just a few simple ingredients from your kitchen and bathroom. This mix leaves out the toxic skin irritants and allows you and your family to breathe easy without having to worry about what you are inhaling as you make your windows sparkle.

2 cups distilled water
½ cup white vinegar
½ cup isopropyl alcohol
20 drops lemon essential oil

1. In a large spray bottle, combine the water, vinegar, alcohol, and essential oil and shake vigorously.
2. To use, spray on windows and mirrors, then wipe away with a clean cloth.
3. Store in a cool, dark place indefinitely and shake well before each use.

Tip: Because essential oils are not water-soluble, it is important that you shake mixtures using distilled water as a base before each use to redistribute the oils throughout the liquid.

Toilet Cleaner

MAKES	PREP TIME
3 to 4 uses	5 minutes

Many commercial toilet bowl cleaners contain chemicals that kill bacteria and viruses, but there is an easy way to get your toilet bowl clean without the harsh abrasives. While the toilet may be one of the dirtiest places in your house, this blend of salt, vinegar, and baking soda is effective in removing tough stains, and the essential oils help kill germs and bacteria lurking in the bowl. This simple mixture will provide three to four toilet cleanings. Feel free to double the recipe's baking soda and salt to have on hand for a longer time, but be sure to add more essential oils before using if the scent has dissipated between uses.

- 1 cup white vinegar
- ½ teaspoon lemon essential oil, divided
- ½ teaspoon tea tree essential oil, divided
- ½ cup baking soda
- ¼ cup coarse salt

1. In a spray bottle, combine the vinegar, ¼ teaspoon of lemon essential oil, and ¼ teaspoon of tea tree essential oil. Close the lid and shake well to mix. Spray the toilet bowl, seat, and handle with the spray.
2. In a small jar, combine the baking soda, salt, and remaining ¼ teaspoon of lemon essential oil, and ¼ teaspoon of tea tree essential oil.
3. Sprinkle the baking soda mixture in the toilet bowl and let sit for about 20 minutes until the bubbling subsides.
4. Using a toilet brush, scrub the toilet and flush. Wipe down the seat and handle with a clean cloth.

Tip: Coarse salt is great for scrubbing surfaces like the toilet bowl that need a little added grit. Use any variety of coarse grain salt you have on hand for this recipe.

Homemade Cleansing Wipes

MAKES
1¼ cups

PREP TIME
5 minutes

If you like disposable wipes for their functionality but aren't a fan of single use products, these general-purpose cleansing wipes are what you need. Using a wide-mouth jar and a small mound of rags or pieces of cloth, you can create your own DIY wipes. After the wipes are used, throw them in the washing machine for a new batch.

¾ cup distilled water

½ cup isopropyl alcohol

1 teaspoon unscented liquid castile soap

10 drops lemon essential oil

5 drops lavender essential oil

1. In a wide-mouth jar, combine the water, alcohol, castile soap, and essential oils. Close the lid securely and shake well to combine.
2. Stuff as many rags, towels, or pieces of cloth that will fit into the jar, firmly secure the lid, and shake. To use, shake the jar to ensure the wipes are moistened, then remove a cloth and wipe the surface clean.
3. When the jar is empty, launder the cloths and return them to the jar, mixing more sanitizing solution as needed.

Tip: There are many companies that sell reusable flannel and cotton wipes (and containers to hold them) for the purpose of making homemade products like this one that cut down on single-use items. Look online to shop the different options or cut up an old T-shirt or other absorbent material into rag-size pieces to use as wipes. If you wish to buy premade wipes, Marley's Monsters is a great source for reusable wipes.

Room Refreshing Spray

MAKES
½ cup

PREP TIME
5 minutes

There are a ton of room spray products on the market, but they can be problematic to people with allergies and may adversely affect many systems of the body. This simple mix is natural and provides a lovely floral scent, without the chemicals. Play around with your favorite scents to create different combinations that suit you.

½ cup distilled water

1 tablespoon witch hazel

30 drops lavender essential oil

1. In a small spray bottle using a small funnel, combine the water, witch hazel, and essential oil. Close the lid and shake to mix well. Spray 3 to 5 times in the air of a room as needed.
2. Store in a cool, dark location indefinitely and shake well before each use to disperse the oils.

Tip: Some other great essential oils that work well to refresh a room include orange, rosemary, peppermint, and cinnamon.

Odor Remover for Carpet

MAKES	PREP TIME
2 cups	5 minutes

Baking soda is used here for its alkaline odor-absorbing qualities, along with purifying oils, which can work to stop odor-producing bacteria in their tracks. Be sure to let the powder sit on the carpet for at least an hour before vacuuming so that it can break through the odors. You can even help it along by working it into the fibers of the carpet so that it can fight odors right at the source.

- 2 cups baking soda
- 15 drops lavender essential oil
- 10 drops tea tree essential oil

1. In a bowl, thoroughly combine the baking soda and essential oils.
2. To use, sprinkle on the carpet and let sit for 1 to 2 hours. Vacuum thoroughly until all the baking soda is vacuumed up.
3. Store any remaining mixture in a tightly sealed mason jar in a cool, dark location indefinitely.

Tip: You can make a shaker top for a mason jar by using an awl or drill to poke holes in the metal and affixing the lid as usual. Just be sure to close the jar with a solid lid for storage so that the scent remains strong. There are also many commercially available mason jar lids with holes in them for shaking different food items, and these make a perfectly good substitute instead. Be sure that children and pets are not allowed on the carpet while the powder sits on it and for up to an hour after vacuuming, as the powder can be irritating to their sensitive systems.

Floor Cleaner Concentrate

MAKES
1½ cups

PREP TIME
5 minutes

Many commercial cleaners affect indoor air quality, and floor cleaners are one of the worst offenders, as they are generally very heavily scented. This cleaner features a light lemon scent and cuts through grease and grime to leave your floors just as clean without the harsh chemicals. Be sure to spot-test this in an inconspicuous spot on your floor before use; it is not recommended for wood floors, as it can remove the finish.

½ cup isopropyl alcohol
½ cup white vinegar
½ cup unscented dish soap
1 teaspoon lemon essential oil

1. In a glass jar, combine the alcohol, vinegar, soap, and essential oil. Cover with a lid (if using a metal lid, place a piece of wax paper in between the jar and lid to create a barrier between the metal and liquid to prevent rusting) and shake well to combine.
2. To use, shake vigorously to mix, then pour 2 tablespoons to ¼ cup in a bucket and fill with hot water. Mop floors with the solution.
3. Store in a cool, dark place indefinitely. Shake well before each use.

Tip: While this will store indefinitely, the lemon scent will fade over time. If you don't smell it any longer after storing, add more lemon essential oil, as needed.

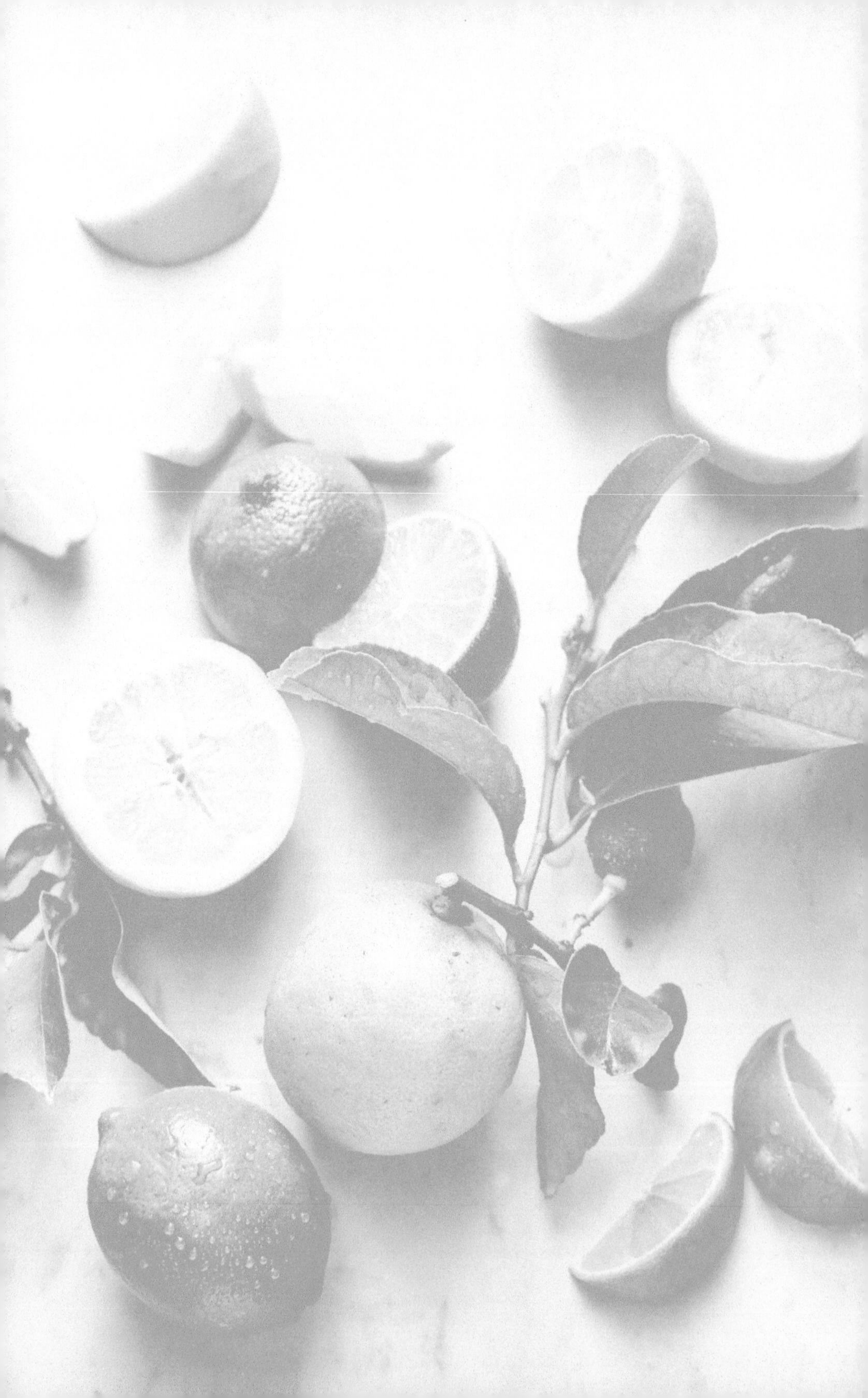

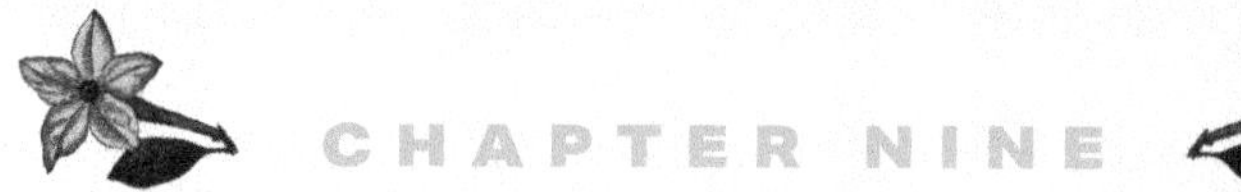

CHAPTER NINE

Helpful Remedies for Common Health Issues

Many of us are used to scooting to the local drugstore and purchasing some of the familiar and well-advertised over-the-counter medicines to address aches, pains, gas, bloating, sniffles, and reflux without knowing the potential damage that long-term use of these items may have on our microbial community. Too often these meds mask the symptoms, which while helpful in the short term, can disrupt our microbial habitat over time. The following recipes are some alternatives for you to try that can help address various symptoms naturally using food (or scents) as therapeutic agents. While research on the effectiveness of the following remedies may be in early stages, none of them is likely to cause any adverse reaction, and they may set you on a whole new course of self-healing methods. Experiment and see what works for your body. Of course, if you are in serious discomfort, please heed the advice of your doctor and take care of yourself.

DIY Mouth Wash (Bad Breath or Gingivitis)

MAKES
1 cup

PREP TIME
5 minutes

Antibacterial ingredients in commercial mouthwashes can eliminate both the good and bad bacteria in the mouth. Because the mouth is the start of our digestive tract, its microbiome health is an important component in healthy digestion. Aloe vera juice can help fight inflammation, and baking soda can assist in fighting bad breath in this natural blend.

½ cup distilled water
½ cup aloe vera juice
1 teaspoon baking soda
1 drop peppermint essential oil
Pinch sea salt

1. In a small jar or bottle, combine the water and aloe vera juice. Add the baking soda, essential oil, and salt. Close the lid and shake well to combine.
2. To use, pour about a tablespoon of the mouthwash into a cup and sip without swallowing. Swish the mouthwash around in your mouth for 20 seconds, then spit.
3. Store in the refrigerator for up to 3 weeks. Shake well before each use to ensure it's well mixed.

Ingredient tip: Aloe vera juice is the liquid extracted from the aloe vera plant. Find it at health food stores or online. Look for pure, organic 100 percent aloe vera juice for the best quality.

Belly Soothing Kudzu Broth (Intestinal Support)

MAKES	PREP TIME	COOK TIME
2 cups	5 minutes	15 minutes

Kudzu is a tonifying herb used in Chinese medicine to relieve pain, ease digestive disorders, and treat diarrhea, colds, headaches, and more. An anti-inflammatory and antimicrobial chalklike powder derived from the plant's root, kudzu is often used as a thickener in cooking, similar to arrowroot flour, and can be made into this tasty broth to provide intestinal support.

2 cups water

1 tablespoon kudzu root powder

1½ teaspoons umeboshi paste

1 teaspoon tamari

1 teaspoon grated fresh ginger root or ginger powder

1. In a small saucepan, whisk the water and kudzu well before heating. Bring to a boil over medium heat, reduce the heat, and simmer for about 5 minutes, until the mixture begins to thicken.
2. Stir in the umeboshi paste, tamari, and ginger and continue to simmer for about 10 more minutes, being careful not to boil.
3. Remove from the heat and serve hot.

Ingredient tip: Umeboshi is a pickled, tart Japanese plum that is served as a condiment both for its intense flavor and health-promoting properties, as it is thought to be a digestive aid. Look for the paste in Japanese markets or order it online. Kudzu root powder is available at health food stores, herb shops, and online.

Golden Milk (Anti-Inflammatory)

MAKES	PREP TIME	COOK TIME
1½ cups	2 minutes	5 minutes

Similar in appearance to ginger, turmeric is a knobby root with vibrant orange flesh. It is a powerful antioxidant and is among the highest-known sources of beta-carotene. The yellow pigment in turmeric, curcumin, is a natural anti-inflammatory, which coupled with ginger's similar properties, makes a simple drink that packs in nutrition and healing support. Enjoy a mug daily for optimal anti-inflammatory benefit.

- 1½ cups unsweetened plain almond, hemp, or coconut milk
- 1½ teaspoons ground turmeric
- 1 teaspoon honey, maple syrup, or agave syrup
- ¼ teaspoon ground ginger, cardamom, or cinnamon
- Pinch freshly ground black pepper

1. In a saucepan, combine the milk, turmeric, honey, ginger, and pepper. Bring to a simmer over medium heat, being careful not to boil.
2. Using an immersion blender or stand blender, blend the milk for 30 seconds, until frothy. Serve hot.

Ingredient tip: While black pepper may seem like an odd choice in a sweet beverage, be sure not to skip it. The pepper provides a complementary flavor and plays a role in making the curcumin in the turmeric more bioavailable, meaning that it helps make it more easily absorbed by your body.

Ginger Tea Tonic (Heartburn Relief)

MAKES	PREP TIME	COOK TIME
1½ cups	5 minutes	10 minutes

Ginger is a perfect ingredient in a digestive tonic, as it can help alleviate acidity and other gastrointestinal irritations like heartburn. Instead of reaching for an antacid, try this brew first. The ginger can reduce inflammation in the body, which may work to relieve the symptoms of acid reflux, as well as other ailments like colds, flu, and even motion sickness. Serve it hot with lemon juice for a soothing and warming drink that supports healthy detoxification.

- 1½ cups water
- 2 inches fresh ginger root, peeled and chopped
- 2 tablespoons freshly squeezed lemon juice
- 2 teaspoons honey

1. In a small saucepan, bring the water to a boil and add the ginger. Turn off the heat and let the ginger steep for 10 minutes.
2. Press the ginger with the back of a spoon to extract as much liquid as possible. Then, using a wire-mesh strainer, strain the liquid into a mug and discard the ginger root.
3. Add the lemon juice and honey. Stir well and drink hot.

Ingredient tip: Ginger can help alleviate symptoms of gastrointestinal irritation when taken in small doses, but overuse can have the opposite effect by irritating the digestive system. When steeping in a tea like this, ginger is entirely safe for regular consumption. For even more bite, grate the ginger to extract more of its juices in the drink.

Fire Cider (Immune Support)

MAKES	PREP TIME
about 2 cups	20 minutes, plus 1 month steeping time

This spicy, pungent cider is loaded with all the right stuff you need to alleviate sinus congestion, aid digestion, and keep colds and flus at bay. A folk remedy used for generations, the end product can be served on its own or mixed into a drink or other recipe for added flavor and benefit. Using a mixture of immune-supporting ginger, horseradish, onion, garlic, turmeric, and jalapeño peppers, this remedy gets your blood flowing with its bold flavors and may help prevent sickness from taking hold. Whip up a batch of this before flu season so that it is ready when the sniffles come on.

- ½ cup chopped fresh ginger root
- ½ cup chopped fresh horseradish root
- 1 small yellow onion, chopped
- ¼ cup coarsely chopped garlic
- ¼ cup coarsely chopped turmeric root or 1 tablespoon turmeric powder
- 3 jalapeño peppers, chopped
- Grated zest and juice of 1 lemon
- 2 to 3 cups unfiltered apple cider vinegar

1. In a quart-size mason jar or other glass jar, combine the ginger, horseradish, onion, garlic, turmeric, jalapeños, and lemon juice and zest. Pour the vinegar over top of the aromatics to cover.
2. Close the jar with a plastic lid or place a piece of parchment paper under the metal lid to prevent the vinegar from coming in contact with the metal. Shake the jar well to combine.
3. Store in a cool, dark location for 1 month, shaking briefly daily to mix.
4. After 1 month, using a mesh strainer set over a bowl, strain the vinegar from the solids. Transfer the strained vinegar to a clean jar and store in the refrigerator for up to 3 months.
5. Take 1 to 2 tablespoons daily on its own or mixed into water at the first sign of a cold and repeat every 3 or 4 hours until resolved, or take 1 tablespoon per day as a preventive. If desired, stir it into another liquid to serve.

Congee (Digestive Support)

SERVES	PREP TIME	COOK TIME
5	10 minutes	3 to 8 hours

Rice porridge, congee, and jook are all names for this long-simmered soup enjoyed around the world in many different forms. Popular in Chinese medicine, it can be customized to support specific health issues, provide ongoing digestive support, and help assist in recovery from illness. Best of all, it can be made in a slow cooker, so it can simmer away while you're asleep or at work.

- 4 cups water or stock, plus additional as needed
- ½ cup white or brown rice
- 1 (2-inch) piece kombu seaweed
- 1 teaspoon minced fresh ginger root
- ½ teaspoon sea salt
- 1 cup chopped cooked chicken breast or cubed tofu
- 2 scallions, white and green parts, thinly sliced, separated

1. In a soup pot or slow cooker, combine the water, rice, seaweed, ginger, and salt. Bring to a boil over high heat, then reduce the heat to low and very slowly simmer for at least 3 hours or up to 8 hours, stirring occasionally. Add additional water, if necessary.
2. Prior to serving, add the chicken and the white parts of the scallions and cook for 5 more minutes, or until the chicken is warmed through. Season to taste and serve, garnished with the scallion greens.

Variation tip: Add a teaspoon of tamari to the congee to serve, if desired, for additional flavor.

CocoBanana Elixir (Diarrhea Remedy)

SERVES 2

PREP TIME 5 minutes

Carob is known to help with diarrhea in infants, while underripe bananas can be a powerful diarrhea remedy. Coconut water helps replace electrolytes, and mint helps with spasms. Combine all four, and you have a mini powerhouse that provides nutrition, replenishes fluids, and is loaded with flavor. The color of the final product may not be pleasing to all, so feel free to present in a festive glass, or one with a lid.

2 underripe bananas

1 cup coconut water

1 teaspoon carob powder

2 to 4 drops peppermint extract or 2 to 3 fresh mint leaves, finely chopped

2 mint leaves, for garnish

1. In a blender, combine the banana, coconut water, carob powder, and peppermint extract and process until smooth. Add more coconut water for a thinner liquid, if desired.
2. Garnish with a mint leaf. Serve immediately.

Ingredient tip: Look for green bananas when making this elixir. When still unripe and firm, bananas are astringent and can provide diarrhea and colitis relief. However, when ripe and sweet, they are more easily digested and, conversely, are used to treat constipation.

Oatmeal Bath (Dry Itchy Skin, Eczema)

MAKES
about ½ cup

PREP TIME
10 minutes

Your skin is the largest organ on your body. Treating it right without the use of harsh ingredients is key to your microbiome health. This simple bath is a classic remedy to soothe itchy, dry skin and can be made in minutes. The chamomile tea can help support skin irritations, soothe muscles, and even possibly promote healthy sleep, so enjoy this before bedtime for the best results.

2 or 3 chamomile tea bags

¼ cup old fashioned rolled oats

2 tablespoons baking soda

1 tablespoon coconut oil

1. Bring a few cups of water to a boil and turn off the heat. Place the tea bags in the water and steep for 10 minutes.
2. Meanwhile, in a blender, blend the oats for about 1 minute until they become a fine powder with no visible oat pieces.
3. Transfer the oats to a small bowl and mix with the baking soda.
4. Run a warm bath and place the oat powder and baking soda mixture in the water, along with the coconut oil and steeped tea. Mix well to disperse the oil. Soak for 15 to 20 minutes.

Preparation tip: The powder should be ground fine enough and dispersed in the water well enough that it shouldn't create a problem in your drain. However, if you are concerned, place the oats in a satchel in the bath water and close with a string, skipping the step of processing them in the blender.

Garlic in Honey (Antiviral, Cold Support)

MAKES	PREP TIME
1 cup	15 minutes, plus 1 month to ferment

Get this recipe going in the fall to have on hand for winter flu season, and you will be glad you did. Using just two ingredients, this is a simple remedy that tastes great. Garlic is antibacterial and may support the body in fighting influenza and can even reduce fever by increasing perspiration. Honey soothes the stomach and lungs, making it a great partner with garlic to support immune health. Raw honey is rich in antioxidants, has antibacterial and antifungal properties, and may provide relief for both a sore throat and digestive issues.

- 2 heads fresh garlic, separated into cloves
- 1 cup raw honey

1. Sterilize a pint-size jar by submerging it in a pot of boiling water for 10 minutes. Use tongs to carefully remove the jar and set it aside.
2. Using a small knife, make an incision on the curved side of each clove of garlic, remove the skins, and cut off the root ends. Using a clean kitchen towel or paper towel, dry the garlic cloves well.
3. Pack the garlic into the sanitized jar, pour the honey over the garlic cloves, stir well, and loosely cover the jar with a lid.
4. Set the jar in a cool location and flip daily to coat the garlic in honey. You can use the honey after 2 to 3 days and eat the garlic after 1 month. Dissolve 1 to 2 teaspoons of the honey in hot water before bed at the onset of a cold and as needed throughout. Eat the garlic after 1 month on its own, as the flavor mellows considerably.

Variation tip: As the garlic ferments, the moisture from it is released into the honey, thinning it out and making a tasty syrup that doesn't have to be used just when you're sick. Try it with cold water as a refreshing beverage, or even in a cocktail.

Bone Broth

MAKES	PREP TIME	COOK TIME
8 cups	10 minutes	7 to 24 hours

Bone broth is one of the easiest things you can make to support your overall health. This simple recipe may help with issues with intestinal permeability and provide support for your joints, all for very little effort. Simply throw the ingredients in a stock pot and let them simmer to break down the collagen and gelatin in the bones that may help assist in healing your body from the inside out. Use high-quality organic and/or humanely raised chickens when possible.

1 whole chicken

4 quarts water

1 large yellow onion, halved

2 carrots, coarsely chopped

3 celery stalks, coarsely chopped

1 tablespoon apple cider vinegar

1. In a large stock pot, combine the chicken, water, onion, carrots, celery, and vinegar. Bring to a boil over high heat, skimming off any scum that rises to the surface.
2. Reduce the heat, cover, and simmer for 1 hour. Remove the chicken from the broth and let cool over a colander set over a bowl, while keeping the broth simmering.
3. When cool enough to handle, remove the chicken from the carcass and return the carcass to the pot. Reserve the chicken for use in other recipes.
4. Continue to simmer the bones and broth for an additional 6 to 24 hours, until reduced by half and darkened.
5. Using a wire-mesh strainer, strain the broth into a storage container. Let cool, remove the fat from the broth, and refrigerate.

Preparation tip: This recipe will produce an extremely flavorful bone broth and enough chicken for several meals. Chop or shred the chicken and portion it into meal-size servings in airtight containers for future recipes. Refrigerate for three to five days or freeze for up to three months.

Detox Tonic

MAKES	PREP TIME	COOK TIME
1½ cups	1 minute	10 minutes

Dandelions may be a pest in the yard, but when it comes to the body, they have historically been a natural remedy for a variety of ailments. The leaves and roots of the dandelion are consumed for their potential tonifying effect on the liver, stomach, kidneys, and spleen. This, combined with the gut-soothing properties of bone broth and the digestive support of mint, creates a warming blend that can help the liver jump-start its important work.

- 1½ cups Bone Broth (page 139)
- 2 mint sprigs
- 1 dandelion root tea bag

1. In a saucepan, heat the bone broth over medium heat until simmering.
2. In a mug, muddle the mint leaves with a pestle. Pour the broth over the leaves. Add the tea bag and let steep for 5 to 10 minutes. Remove the tea bag, pressing against the side of the mug with a spoon to remove as much tea as possible. Serve hot.

Ingredient tip: Dandelion root can be used to combat many ailments, including those affecting the digestive system. However, some people are allergic to it, and it can interact with certain medications. Consult with a doctor before use if taking prescription medications.

Thyroid Support Tonic

MAKES	PREP TIME	COOK TIME
1½ cups	1 minute	20 minutes

Iodine is necessary in the diet to support normal thyroid function. Seaweeds such as kelp and dulse are some of the best natural sources for iodine and bring a great nutritional boost of other minerals to your diet. This flavorful blend is simple yet effective in providing thyroid support.

- 1½ cups Bone Broth (page 139)
- 2 tablespoons kelp or dulse flakes
- Pinch sea salt

1. In a small saucepan, heat the broth over medium heat. Add the kelp and salt and simmer for 10 to 15 minutes.
2. Pour into a mug and drink hot.

Ingredient tip: Kelp should be eaten in moderation and avoided altogether for people with hyperthyroidism or those with active autoimmune thyroid issues. Be sure to select an organic variety that has been tested for arsenic, as heavy metals can be absorbed into sea vegetables. Avoid all concentrated kelp and seaweed products in pill and powder forms, as they can have excessively high levels of iodine, which can be harmful to the body.

Measurement Conversions

	US STANDARD	US STANDARD (OUNCES)	METRIC (APPROXIMATE)
VOLUME EQUIVALENTS (LIQUID)	2 tablespoons	1 fl. oz.	30 mL
	¼ cup	2 fl. oz.	60 mL
	½ cup	4 fl. oz.	120 mL
	1 cup	8 fl. oz.	240 mL
	1½ cups	12 fl. oz.	355 mL
	2 cups or 1 pint	16 fl. oz.	475 mL
	4 cups or 1 quart	32 fl. oz.	1 L
	1 gallon	128 fl. oz.	4 L
VOLUME EQUIVALENTS (DRY)	⅛ teaspoon	—	0.5 mL
	¼ teaspoon	—	1 mL
	½ teaspoon	—	2 mL
	¾ teaspoon	—	4 mL
	1 teaspoon	—	5 mL
	1 tablespoon	—	15 mL
	¼ cup	—	59 mL
	⅓ cup	—	79 mL
	½ cup	—	118 mL
	⅔ cup	—	156 mL
	¾ cup	—	177 mL
	1 cup	—	235 mL
	2 cups or 1 pint	—	475 mL
	3 cups	—	700 mL
	4 cups or 1 quart	—	1 L
	½ gallon	—	2 L
	1 gallon	—	4 L
WEIGHT EQUIVALENTS	½ ounce	—	15 g
	1 ounce	—	30 g
	2 ounces	—	60 g
	4 ounces	—	115 g
	8 ounces	—	225 g
	12 ounces	—	340 g
	16 ounces or 1 pound	—	455 g

	FAHRENHEIT (°F)	CELSIUS (°C) (APPROXIMATE)
OVEN TEMPERATURES	250°F	120°C
	300°F	150°C
	325°F	180°C
	375°F	190°C
	400°F	200°C
	425°F	220°C
	450°F	230°C

Resources

Hungry for more information? See the following recommendations for a few additional resources that might benefit you.

Books

Follow Your Gut: How the Ecosystem in Your Gut Determines Your Health, Mood, and More by Rob Knight: This fairly short book written by a scientist working with the American Gut Project gives a great overview of some of the basics of this topic.

The Mind-Gut Connection: How the Hidden Conversation Within Our Bodies Impacts Our Mood, Our Choices, and Our Overall Health by Emeran Mayer: This book helps us understand the relationship between our gut and brain and what to do about it.

Websites

American Gut Project, humanfoodproject.com/americangut/: This website is a place where you can actually take part in the research occurring around the gut microbiome by sending in a de-identified stool sample and comparing your microbial population to others around the country.

The Gut Microbiota for Health, gutmicrobiotaforhealth.com: This site is an incredible resource that will keep you up to date on the latest research around the gut microbiome and inform you about its yearly world summit.

The NIH Human Microbiome Project, hmpdacc.org: This project led by the National Institutes of Health is keeping track of research around the connection between the human microbiome and a variety of diseases.

Articles

"Plant-Based Diets and the Gut Microbiota" by Carrie Dennett, todaysdietitian.com/newarchives/0718p36.shtml: Although written for dietitians, this short article provides an excellent overview of ways to eat to optimize gut function.

"Probiotics: What You Need To Know," https://www.nccih.nih.gov/health/probiotics-what-you-need-to-know: This is an excellent general article about probiotics put out by a division of the NIH called the National Center for Complementary and Integrative Health.

"The Influence of Soil on Immune Health," https://www.the-scientist.com/news-opinion/the-influence-of-soil-on-human-health-66885: This is a great read on a hot new topic that is bound to get more play in the next few years—how our exposure to microbes in our environment is critical to human health.

Podcasts

"Microbiome: The Essential Ecosystem in Your Belly" from Mary's Nutrition Show," marypurdy.co/microbiome: This podcast episode from yours truly gives some tips on improving your microbiome status with diet and lifestyle.

Top Podcasts About the Gut Microbiome and Digestive Health, atlasbiomed.com/blog/best-gut-microbiome-podcasts: This is a fantastic list of a variety of podcasts on the microbiome. There should be a topic here that suits your fancy!

Videos

"Exploring the Invisible Universe That Lives On Us—And In Us," npr.org/sections/health-shots/2013/11/01/242361826/exploring-the-invisible-universe-that-lives-on-us-and-in-us: This five-minute animated video takes you through a simple lesson on how the gut microbiome develops.

"How the Food You Eat Affects Your Gut" ed.ted.com/lessons/how-the-food-you-eat-affects-your-gut-shilpa-ravella: This short, delightful, and easy-to-understand animated video provides a peek into how your microbes respond to the food you eat.

Companies

Labdoor, labdoor.com: This is an independent company that tests supplements and is a great way to ensure that supplements you purchase are of high quality.

Microbiome Labs, microbiomelabs.com: Not only is this an excellent supplement company with a trustworthy and effective product, but its website provides educational blogs and webinars, as well as information about clinical trials and upcoming conferences.

Cookbooks

Fresh and Fermented by Julie O'Brien: This cookbook written by the owner of Seattle's fabulous fermented foods company Firefly Kitchens (fireflykitchens.com) provides a variety of recipes that help you include fermented foods into your everyday meals—including your smoothie!

Wild Fermentation: The Flavor, Nutrition, and Craft of Live-Culture Foods by Sandor Katz: This book, written by the famous king of fermentation, is both a history and celebration of fermented and cultured foods and a creative cookbook that has a little something for everyone.

References

Blum, Winfried E.H., Sophie Zechmeister-Boltenstern, and Katharina M. Keiblinger. "Does Soil Contribute to the Human Gut Microbiome?" *Microorganisms* 7, no. 9 (2019): 287. https://doi.org/10.3390/microorganisms7090287.

Carabotti, Marilia, Annunziata Scirocco, Maria Antonietta Maselli, and Carola Severi. "The Gut-Brain Axis: Interactions Between Enteric Microbiota, Central and Enteric Nervous Systems." *Annals of Gastroenterology* 28, no. 2 (2015): 203–209.

Chun, O. K., N. Smith, A. Sacagawa and C. Y. Lee. "Antioxidant Properties of Raw and Processed Cabbages." *International Journal of Food Sciences and Nutrition* 55, no. 3 (2004): 191–199.

Colombo, M., Castilho, N.P.A., Todorov, S. D. et al. "Beneficial Properties of Lactic Acid Bacteria Naturally Present in Dairy Production." *BMC Microbiology* 18, no. 219 (2018). https://doi.org/10.1186/s12866-018-1356-8.

Gorbach, Sherwood L. "Microbiology of the Gastrointestinal Tract." In *Medical Microbiology*, edited by Samuel Baron. Galveston: University of Texas Medical Branch, 1996. https://www.ncbi.nlm.nih.gov/books/NBK7670.

Hansen, M., Meagan A. Rubel, Aubrey G. Bailey, et al. Tishkoff. "Population Structure of Human Gut Bacteria in a Diverse Cohort from Rural Tanzania and Botswana." *Genome Biology* 20, no. 16 (2019). https://doi.org/10.1186/s13059-018-1616-9.

Hills, Ronald D., Benjamin A. Pontefract, Hillary R. Mishcon, et al. "Gut Microbiome: Profound Implications for Diet and Disease." *Nutrients* 11, no. 7 (2019): 1,613. https://doi.org/10.3390/nu11071613.

Li, J., R. Yu, L. Zhang, et al. "Dietary Fructose-Induced Gut Dysbiosis Promotes Mouse Hippocampal Neuroinflammation: A Benefit of Short-Chain Fatty Acids." *Microbiome* 7, no. 1 (2019). https://doi.org/10.1186/s40168-019-0713-7.

Maier, L., M. Pruteanu, M. Kuhn, et al. "Extensive Impact of Non-Antibiotic Drugs on Human Gut Bacteria." *Nature* 555, (2018): 623–628. https://doi.org/10.1038/nature25979.

National Academies of Sciences, Engineering, and Medicine. *Environmental Chemicals, the Human Microbiome, and Health Risk: A Research Strategy*. Washington, DC: The National Academies Press, 2018.

National Institutes of Health. "Bacteria on Skin Boost Immune Cell Function." July 26, 2012. https://www.nih.gov/news-events/nih-research-matters/bacteria-skin-boost-immune-cell-function.

NIH News in Health. "Mouth Microbes: The Helpful and the Harmful." Accessed January 2020. https://newsinhealth.nih.gov/2019/05/mouth-microbes.

Ozdal, Tugba, David A. Sela, Jianbo Xiao, et al. "The Reciprocal Interactions between Polyphenols and Gut Microbiota and Effects on Bioaccessibility." *Nutrients* 8, no. 22 (2016): 78. https://doi.org/10.3390/nu8020078.

Proal, A. D., P. J. Albert, and T. G. Marshall. "The Human Microbiome and Autoimmunity." *Current Opinion in Rheumatology* 25, no. 2 (2013): 234–40. https:doi.org/10.1097/BOR.0b013e32835cedbf.

Quagliani, D., and P. Felt-Gunderson. "Closing America's Fiber Intake Gap: Communication Strategies From a Food and Fiber Summit." *American Journal of Lifestyle Medicine* 11, no. 1 (2015): 80–85. https://doi.org/10.1177/1559827615588079.

Richter, Josef, Vladimir Svozil, Vlastimil Král, Lucie Rajnohová Dobiášová, and Vaclav Vetvicka. "β-glucan Affects Mucosal Immunity in Children with Chronic Respiratory Problems under Physical Stress: Clinical Trials." *Annals of Translational Medicine* 3, no. 4 (2015). https://doi.org/10.3978/j.issn.2305-5839.2015.03.20.

Rodale Institute. "Soil Health." Accessed January 2019. https://rodaleinstitute.org/why-organic/organic-farming-practices/soil-health.

Ruiz-Ojeda, Francisco Javier, Julio Plaza-Díaz, Maria Jose Sáez-Lara, and Angel Gil. "Effects of Sweeteners on the Gut Microbiota: A Review of Experimental Studies and Clinical Trials." *Advances in Nutrition* 10, no. 1 (2019). https://doi.org/10.1093/advances/nmy037.

Schroeder, Bjoern O. "Fight Them or Feed Them: How the Intestinal Mucus Layer Manages the Gut Microbiota." *Gastroenterology Report* 7, no. 1 (2019): 3–12. https://doi.org/10.1093/gastro/goy052.

Singh, R. K., H. W. Chang, D. Yan, K. M. Lee, et al. "Influence of Diet on the Gut Microbiome and Implications for Human Health." *Journal of Translational Medicine* 15, no. 1. https://doi.org/10.1186/s12967-017-1175-y.

Smith, Robert P., Cole Easson, Sarah M. Lyle, Ritishka Kapoor, et al. "Gut Microbiome Diversity Is Associated with Sleep Physiology in Humans." *PLOS One* 14, no. 10 (2019). https://doi.org/10.1371/journal.pone.0222394.

Snopek, Lukas, Jiri Mlcek, Lenka Sochorova, Mojmir Baron, et al. “Contribution of Red Wine Consumption to Human Health Protection.” *Molecules* 23, no. 7 (2018): 1,684. https://doi.org/10.3390/molecules23071684.

Terciolo, C., M. Dapoigny , and F. Andre. “Beneficial Effects of *Saccharomyces boulardii* CNCM I-745 on Clinical Disorders Associated with Intestinal Barrier Disruption.” *Clinical and Experimental Gastroenterology* 12, no. 1 (2019): 67–82. https://doi.org/10.2147/CEG.S181590.

Index

W

Y

Z

Acknowledgments

Thank you to the light and love of my life, Keith, who patiently listens to me frequently ooze on about fiber. He always has a smile of gratitude and a heartfelt "It's good!" or "It's hitting the spot!" to the creative meals I sometimes put in front of him, especially if he knows they will make his bacteria rejoice.

Thank you to my incredibly loving mom and dad who have forever encouraged and championed my ongoing education, career choices, and various ventures—even if it means a long conversation where they stare blankly at me while I try to explain the meaning of "butyrate."

Thank you to my smart and soulful colleagues in the Dietitians in Integrative and Functional Medicine group whose bacteria-rich articles I have devoured, digestive-focused webinars I have watched, and heartfelt support I feel no matter what project I seem to find myself working on.

Thank you to my fellow coaches, clinicians, and researchers at Arivale who taught me a great deal about the ins and outs of the microbiome, especially the brilliant Ohad Manor who always welcomed additional questions about bacteria—especially if he could also quote his favorite *Seinfeld* episodes at some point during the conversation. And thanks to all the Arivale clients who donated their stool samples so that we could better understand the microbiome and get practice saying "firmicutes" and "verrucomicrobia" hundreds of times.

Thank you to Katherine Green who helped to develop the majority of the recipes contained herein. You created a bevy of delectable dishes and inspired me to clean my tub with baking soda.

Finally, thank you to the folks at Callisto Media, especially Gurvinder Gandu, who reached out and gave me this opportunity to share my knowledge, offer insights, and maintain my writing voice and sense of humor throughout.

About the Author

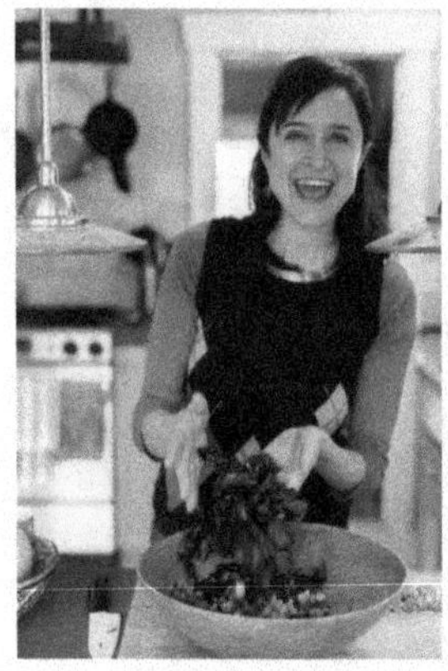

Mary Purdy, MS, RDN, is an integrative and eco-minded dietitian who holds a master's degree in clinical nutrition from Bastyr University, where she has been adjunct faculty since 2015. She has provided nutrition and lifestyle counseling for over 12 years, has given more than 100 nutrition workshops, and speaks nationally at health and nutrition conferences on the topics of both nutritional and environmental health. She is the cocreator of the revised "Environmental Toxins, Exposure, and Elimination" module of the Certificate of Training Program offered by The Academy Center for Lifelong Learning and coauthored the "Diet Appendix for The Anti-Inflammatory Diet" chapter for the 14th and 15th editions of *Krause's Food & the Nutrition Care Process*. She hosts the podcast *Mary's Nutrition Show*, is the author of the book *Serving the Broccoli Gods*, and is a tireless advocate for a more sustainable food system that supports our environment and works to mitigate climate change.